CREATING A VISION FOR HEALTH

DON EASTON

Copyright © 2024 Donald T Easton

All rights reserved. Except for the quotation of small passages for the purposes of criticism or review, no part of this publication may be reproduced, stored in a retrieval system or transmitted in any form or by any means, electronic, mechanical, photocopying, recording, scanning or otherwise, without the permission in writing of the author.

Without in any way limiting the author's and publisher's exclusive rights under copyright, any use of this publication to 'train' generative artificial intelligence (AI) technologies to generate text is expressly prohibited. The author reserves all rights to license uses of this work for generative AI training and development of machine learning language models.

Although the author and publisher have made every effort to ensure that the information in this book was correct at press time, the author and publisher do not assume and hereby disclaim any liability to any party for any loss, damage, or disruption caused by errors or omissions, whether such errors or omissions result from negligence, accident, or any other cause.

Scripture quotations marked NLT are taken from the Holy Bible, New Living Translation, copyright ©1996, 2004, 2015 by Tyndale House Foundation. Used by permission of Tyndale House Publishers, Carol Stream, Illinois 60188. All rights reserved.

Scripture quotations marked TPT are from The Passion Translation®. Copyright © 2017, 2018, 2020 by Passion & Fire Ministries, Inc. Used by permission. All rights reserved. ThePassionTranslation.com.

Scripture quotations marked NIV are taken from the Holy Bible, New International Version®, NIV®. Copyright © 1973, 1978, 1984, 2011 by Biblica, Inc.™ Used by permission of Zondervan. All rights reserved worldwide. www.zondervan.com The "NIV" and "New International Version" are trademarks registered in the United States Patent and Trademark Office by Biblica, Inc.™

Scripture quotations marked MSG are taken from THE MESSAGE, copyright © 1993, 2002, 2018 by Eugene H. Peterson. Used by permission of NavPress, represented by Tyndale House Publishers. All rights reserved.

Kindle Edition, License Notes

This eBook is licensed for your personal enjoyment only. This eBook may not be re-sold or given away to other people. If you would like to share this book with another person, please purchase an additional copy for each recipient. If you're reading this book and did not purchase it, or it was not purchased for your use only, then please return to your favourite eBook retailer and purchase your own copy. Thank you for respecting the hard work of this author.

ISBN: 978-1-7635474-0-7

Imprint: Independently published
Cover design and layout: Joshua Easton

CONTENTS

Foreword ii

The Search for Health..viii

Biblical Basis for Health..12

What is the Health of a Christian Leader Assessment? 18

How to Best Use This Tool...26

Vital Spirituality...36

Thriving Relationships 59

Emotional Intelligence...82

Sustainable Life 104

Reduced Risk 124

Conclusion 138

ACKNOWLEDGMENTS

Thank you to my wife, Adrienne, my children, their spouses and children. Your love and support have been my light in the dark.

Thank you to my life-changing mentor, Dr Keith Farmer, whose constant questions, "How are you and Jesus? How are your key relationships? How's your emotional tank? Is your world sustainable? Where are you at risk?" helped shape the five core competencies. Your mentoring was transformative.

Thanks to Dr Chris Adams, Biola University, who led the 2016 Health of a Christian Leader class and presented his scientific research in well-being. Thanks for becoming a friend and helping on the journey.

Thanks to Dr Bob Logan, my professional coach since 2018, whose encouragement, support and guidance has been invaluable in developing these ideas and transforming them into a guide for others. I deeply appreciate our friendship and your transformative coaching.

Thanks Prof. Chuck Ridley for your key qualitative research guidance.

Thank you to Cecelia Meserve for bringing order and readability to my words, research and learning with your wonderful word craft.

To my wife, Adrienne, for your editing prowess from my first theological paper to editing this latest book.

Foreword

Robert E. Logan

If you are a Christian leader looking to avoid—or recover from—burnout, this is the resource for you. Don Easton has put together the full package of assessment tool and resource guide to help you wherever you find yourself on the journey of holistic and Spirit-empowered health.

I first met Don Easton when he audited a class I was teaching at Fuller Seminary. He asked me to lunch, and our professional and personal relationship grew from there. I've seldom met anyone as passionate about the importance of holistic health for ministry leaders as Don. The reason for that passion is his own experience of ministry burnout and his journey back toward health, and that is the subject he writes about in this book.

I have journeyed alongside him as his coach for a number of years now and have walked him through his development of the various profiles included in Creating a Vision of Health. Don is a classic example of 2 Corinthians 1:3-4 (NIV) *Praise be to the God and Father of our Lord Jesus Christ, the Father of compassion and the God of all comfort, who comforts us in all our troubles, so that we can comfort those in any trouble with the comfort we ourselves receive from God.*

Here is a person who cares deeply and is a lifelong learner. His insights and ministry flow out of personal experience—now he has the calling and commitment to empower and equip others to be able to do this important work as well.

Yet the contents here are not just autobiographical. They are also principle-based and research-based. I can tell you that Don has done his homework, putting in the time and thought necessary for a project of this scope and collaborating with professional researchers to determine the validity of his assessment tool. Here Don has created a system of accurate measurement by which individual leaders can assess, grow, then periodically reassess.

Creating a Vision of Health is jam-packed with practical tools for application. Not only can the online survey he developed be taken to capture where a leader is on the burnout scale at any point in time, but he has also thoughtfully included reflection questions to help people process their assessment results effectively and identify a personalised growth plan tailored uniquely to that person.

The need for this book has never been greater. It would serve as a great resource for whole denominations and networks to use on an ongoing basis as a means to track and improve the holistic health of their pastors, planters, and other ministry leaders. Only once we know our starting point can we cultivate the places where healing happens.

Don embodies the kind of caring that life flows out of. That's what impresses me about him and why I'm so privileged to walk alongside him as he makes this significant contribution to the Kingdom of God.

Read it, digest it, use it… for yourself and for others. It will make a significant difference as we raise up and support more healthy leaders for the Kingdom of God.

Dr Robert E. Logan (Bob)
Author: *The Discipleship Difference* (2016) Amazon

ENDORSEMENTS

Dr. Don Easton has written an indispensable field manual for ministry leaders. Creating a Vision for Health is a premium and practical guide to help you develop competencies needed to be a healthy Christian leader. By applying the wisdom contained in Creating a Vision for Health, you will elevate your leadership resiliency, longevity and influence. Read this book. Apply the principles. Enjoy ministry more!

Dr. Wes Beavis
Clinical Psychologist, Newport Beach, California
Author: *Let's Talk about Ministry Burnout* (2019) Powerborn

In his new book, Don Easton presents a vision of healthy Christian leadership. His conclusions are based on decades of Christian leadership and his own experience of burnout and recovery, as well as professionally validated research. These pages are packed with practical insights, reflective questions and helpful resources. Don describes five 'gauges' of concrete behavioural expressions which give a snapshot of what is currently going on inside a leader. This book is a significant advance toward preventing burnout.

A gift to the Body of Christ and Christian leaders everywhere. Insightful. Practical. Excellent!

Dr Mark Fields
Director of Global & Intercultural Ministry, Vineyard USA Retired

I believe anyone wanting to live a healthy, meaningful, purpose filled life that they love, would benefit from reading Don's book, Creating a Vision for Health. It is a reminder of the importance of health and well-being, and also gives valuable tools to be intentional about building a sustainable life. Don's own experiences, generously shared, encourage readers to seek out key relationships, have good support systems in place, and create margins and boundaries. The excellent reflective questions throughout the book are challenging and thought-provoking. I'm sure that this book will be a valuable resource for many.

Ps Susan Marcuccio
President, Australasian Association of Supervision (AAOS)
National Supervision and Mentoring Director, Chaplaincy Australia
Author: *New Perspectives in Supervision* (2022) Perspective Supervision

In Creating a Vision for Health, Don Easton provides ministry leaders with a guide to assess their well-being and practical tools to take steps towards greater health. Ministry leaders who read and implement the wisdom that Easton shares will be more encouraged, more aware of themselves and others, and more effective in their leadership.

Rev. Dr. Thad Austin
Executive Director of the Common Table Collaborative for
Clergy and Congregational Well-Being.
Author: *Caring for Clergy* (2022) Cascade Books

Combining a steep learning curve from his own (significant) breakdown and academic rigour, Don Easton has crafted an exceptional tool for leaders, that has the potential of saving others the pain and losses of bitter experience. Being a healthy leader is not something we stumble upon, but listening to the wise and godly experience of others can assist us enormously to not fall into the traps so common in passionate and driven people. This book is an excellent signpost to effective, healthy and sustainable leadership; mix it with intention and discipline and you have a way forward. Highly recommended.

Simon McIntyre
C3 Church Global Team
Author: *Joshua – Lessons in the Wilderness* (2023) Amazon

We have known Don for 15 years, as a friend, colleague, a successful pastor, through burnout and now beyond. His perceptions on life and people, and his ability to self-reflect are among many of his attributes. This book is not just for those who have faced the 'edge', but for those who want to live with a healthy mind, soul and rhythm—for leaders and people who want to know how to thrive under pressures. The guides, competencies and tools covered in this book are professionally supported and intensely practical. A unique and a must-read book.

Steve and Lizby Warren
C3 Church Europe Directors
Author: *Devoted* (2023) Amazon

When we think of clergy/leader health, we often think in terms of rescuing leaders from burnout and painful dysfunction. However, in this easily read book, Easton provides a guide for mentor and mentee alike to build resiliency in ministry/leadership before burnout occurs. I envisage this book being used as a resource in both the assessment of leader health and the building of proactive steps to build a healthy leader.
Taking five key competencies of a healthy leader, Easton has given a vision of what a healthy leader looks like. This is no theoretical work. Hammered out on the anvil of many years of pastoral leadership, he provides not only warning signs, but just as importantly, rich descriptions of where leaders can realistically be. As such, this is a hopeful and optimistic book delighting in the magnanimous grace of God. I thoroughly recommend this as engaging reading for every leader at whatever stage of their journey in leadership.

Dr Bruce G Allder,
Asia Pacific Region Education Coordinator, Church of the Nazarene
Senior Lecturer Pastoral Theology and Ministry,
Nazarene Theological College, Brisbane, Australia.

INTRODUCTION

The Search for Health

The role of a leader can take many shapes; a mentor, a guide, a coach, a parental figure, a captain... and more. However, regardless of the title, experience, skillset or background, one thing is always true for leaders: leaders bear responsibility for those they lead. This truth can be a lot to handle at times. Great responsibility often leads to great stress and anxiety. Good leaders care deeply about the people around them, about their role and how they serve others; this can make it difficult to prioritise their own well-being. The world of ministry is fast paced, emotionally involved and socially active. It requires time management, problem solving, delegation and people rearing... among other unique skills. At its heart, ministry is a care-giving profession and there is always more care to give. Many leaders succumb to the pressure of their role and eventually burnout at some point in their life. This in turn, negatively impacts both their career and their homelife.

As a pastor, mentor and leader in the Christian community, I have witnessed a lot of burnout first-hand. I've seen friends who are known to be strong leaders, diligent workers, creative thinkers and resilient problem solvers, find themselves exhausted, depressed and without motivation after years of non-stop, difficult work. I've seen leaders who seemed to be born for this sort of vocation lose their steam and spend years feeling emotionally depleted. The work they once loved and that gave them energy and hope, was now draining them. Eventually, their emotional depletion began to take a toll on their work, their co-workers, their projects and priorities, and eventually trickled outside of the confines of their job to their homes, their families, friends, hobbies and overall health. Ultimately, the whole community and God's mission suffered.

I have experienced severe burnout as a pastor and Christian leader. Thankfully, I was able to come through it stronger with the care and support of the people around me. I was more fortunate than many. It was this experience that made me realise the value of my overall well-being. With the help of many friends in the field, I began to study burnout and what it looks like to live a healthy and balanced life. I reached out to leaders in the field, took classes and seminars on the subject, and eventually became a licensed well-being mentor.

My concept of personal well-being changed completely after my experience, and I realised that my misunderstanding of physical, spiritual and emotional health was a large part of what led me to burnout in the first place. Since this experience, I have begun to see signs of burnout all around me, in different stages, with different symptoms and with varying results. But what could we, as their friends, co-workers and partners, do to help ensure the well-being of those around us? How could we begin to identify the root problems that create burnout? What could we do to stabilise and revitalise our community in a sustainable way? I and many others in my field began to ask, 'What does a healthy Christian leader look like? What competencies do they have that are essential? What principles propel them forward? How do they balance personal life with their work?'

During this time, I began to recognize the areas of health that could be measured and observed. This led to the development of well-being gauges which cover five areas of life—Spiritual, Financial, Emotional, Relational and Physical. While these are not a complete analysis of a person's well-being, observing these five areas can provide a snapshot of health and direction regarding the areas needing attention. You can learn more about the well-being gauges here: https://vervelead.com/gauges

In 2021, I developed the *Health of a Christian Leader Assessment*, once referred to as *Well-Being Q*, with the assistance of several experts. It has been built on the mentoring method of Dr Keith Farmer (author of *Going Deeper to Go Further* and former principal of the Australian College of Ministries) and developed with the expertise of field leaders, Dr Charles Ridley (Professor of Educational Psychology at Texas A&M University) and Dr Robert Logan (Logan Leadership, author of *The Leadership Difference* and *The Discipleship Difference*).

The Health of a Christian Leader Assessment provides a way to evaluate the overall well-being of Christian leaders by highlighting strengths in how they function as well as areas that may need development. It is best used with a mentor to debrief the results. The goal is to create a more complete picture of yourself as a leader. It is not a diagnosis, rather a snapshot of your current self, allowing you to see a path toward increased resilience and a better-balanced life and to become an even more effective leader of your community. Most significantly, the work God has given you will become clearer and more energising. You will feel vitalized and excited to pursue your calling and better equipped to handle the disappointments and frustrations of your work, as well as be more aware of the blessings and successes that surround you.

A Biblical Basis for Health

We are made in God's image; designed to be resilient, strong and healthy. There was no physical or emotional sickness in the Garden of Eden, but now our world is far from perfect... as are we. We fall ill, whether through poor decisions or the nature of the world around us. Fortunately, we are also designed to heal and grow, to learn from our experiences and make changes for the better.

In the Bible, there are many notable moments regarding healing from illness. What comes to mind for most are the abundance of stories where Jesus healed the sick: the crippled man (Mark 2:9-12), the bleeding woman (Matthew 9:20-22), the ten Lepers (Luke 17:12-16), the blind man at the pool (John 9:6-7) and many others. He even brought back several people from the dead. Jesus never shamed anyone for their condition. He understood sickness and took compassion on those experiencing pain, weariness and discomfort. It's evident that Jesus cares about our health and He desires us to be the best versions of ourselves. We can do the same by encouraging others to take care of themselves, even if it is inconvenient. 2 Corinthians 1:4 (TPT) says, *He always comes alongside us to comfort us in every suffering so that we can come alongside those who are in any painful trial. We can bring them this same comfort that God has poured out upon us.* Ultimately, we are helping our entire community by allowing ourselves to be honest about our emotional well-being and our needs and encouraging each other to do the same.

There are also many Biblical accounts of people taking care of their own health. In Galatians 4:13 (TPT) Paul writes, *You are well aware that the reason I stayed among you to preach the good news was because of the poor state of my health.* Here was a man of God watching out for his own health while making the best of his situation. He could have gone on travelling, endangering himself and others, but instead elected to rest and recover. There were benefits of this decision. Paul was able to continue sharing the good news to the Galatians. Taking care of ourselves and each other benefits everyone around and also furthers God's mission.

Throughout the New Testament, we can see moments where even Jesus needed to prioritise His own well-being over the needs of people around Him. After John the Baptist was beheaded, Jesus *withdrew by boat privately to a solitary place.* Matthew 14:13 (NIV). Mark tells the story as well, *Then, because so many people were coming and going that they did not even have a chance to eat, he said to them, "Come with me by yourselves to a quiet place and get some rest".* Mark 6:31 (NIV). Jesus needed to rest, grieve and eat before He could continue His work.

Mark shares an example of Jesus making a difficult decision to leave a town, despite the need that was still present. He knew that the needs of the people were infinite and He did not have time to help everyone. It was better for His mission, and for Himself, to travel through many towns:

> [35] *Before daybreak the next morning, Jesus got up and went out to an isolated place to pray.* [36] *Later Simon and the others went out to find him.* [37] *When they found him, they said, 'Everyone is looking for you.'*
> [38] *But Jesus replied, 'We must go on to other towns as well, and I will preach to them, too. That is why I came.'* [39] *So he travelled throughout the region of Galilee, preaching in the synagogues and casting out demons.*
> Mark 1:35-39 (NLT)

Like Jesus, we need to recognize that our work is only as sustainable as we are. Without rest and proper prioritisation of our tasks, we will burnout before we are finished.

Going through burnout was one of the most difficult times of my life, but I now consider it a blessing. My sickness showed me truths about myself, forced me to slow down and self-reflect, and finally, as I healed, allowed me space to change many bad habits in my life.

There are many self-help books, conferences, podcasts and coaches who will tell you how to achieve a healthy work/life balance. There's a lot of wisdom in these. However, I am writing from the perspective of a Christian leader. My approach to well-being is not only physical, emotional and mental, but also, spiritual. In fact, I believe that our spirituality, our faith in the Lord, is the foundation of our health.

The theology of health is the understanding that well-being flows through a relationship with God. Health is a God-given idea; Jesus spent much of his time on earth healing the sick and crippled. 3 John 1:2 (NLT) reads, *Dear friend, I hope all is well with you and that you are as healthy in body as you are strong in spirit.* The Lord wants his people to experience health and wholeness, peace and abundance. God wants to transform us into the versions of ourselves we were created to be. Romans 12:2 (NIV) tells us, *Do not conform to the pattern of this world, but be transformed by the renewing of your mind. Then you will be able to test and approve what God's will is—his good, pleasing and perfect will.* 2 Corinthians 3:18 (NIV) goes deeper into this transformation saying, *And we all, who with unveiled faces contemplate the Lord's glory, are being transformed into his image with ever-increasing glory, which comes from the Lord, who is the Spirit.*

This transformation is a process of change that is enduring and lasting; it requires deeper and more powerful sources than just our own decisions, will-power and strength. It requires the work of God. The theology of health goes further than just our own well-being. While health starts with us, there is also a calling to be of help to others, and that caring and loving the people around us is part of the holistic picture of health. It is good for our soul to be kind, charitable and loving. It is good for our relationships to learn, grow and give as much as we take. Christian well-being is built on relationships, beginning with our relationship with Jesus and using that to build transformative relationships with others. We were not created to be solitary: we were made to work together, to allow ourselves to be transformed, and then to help those around us transform as well. As Christian leaders, we are beholden to this.

Creating a Vision of Health

What is the Health of a Christian Leader Assessment?

The Health of a Christian Leader Assessment is the profile of a healthy Christian leader— a clear picture of an effective leader. I believe that if I had known what a healthy Christian Leader looked like from the beginning and if I had put intentional effort into discovering how I could achieve that in my own life, I could have avoided burnout. I have spoken to many others who feel the same. The profile shows a holistic view with examples of how strong leaders function in all aspects of their lives.

The areas that most people observe when considering their overall well-being are: 1) Spiritual, 2) Physical, 3) Financial, 4) Emotional and 5) Social. These areas help to illuminate unhealthy habits and red flags. I like to take time each week to reflect on how I am doing within each of these essential areas of my life. However, when considering how to frame the Health of a Christian Leader Assessment, we wanted to go deeper and focus on capabilities of a leader, rather than just areas of life. This way we could highlight behaviours and their roots. After a lot of consideration, we narrowed down the main competencies that are required in all healthy Christian leaders to:

- Vital Spirituality
- Thriving Relationships
- Emotional Intelligence
- Sustainable Life
- Reduced Risk

These five core competencies break down into a set of behavioural expressions. For example, the first behavioural expression for 'Vital Spirituality' is *Aligns identity in Christ with scripture*. We then provide examples for a leader who has a high proficiency in this expression (H), a leader who has a fair proficiency (M) and a leader who has a low proficiency (L). This is to help ground the behavioural expression in actions you may or may not take in your everyday life. The purpose is not to provide a grade or pass judgement, only to give you an idea of where you are currently with this particular behavioural expression. Everyone should have some they are highly proficient in, and everyone will have behavioural expressions that need some work. Being able to see these clearly is the first step.

It's best to take the *Health of a Christian Leader Assessment* before you continue reading to gain insight into your current health.

Then as you read further you'll begin to recognise your own strengths and areas for growth.

I've found that having a well-being mentor is a crucial element to effectively use this profile, and we will encourage the use of a mentor throughout this book. A well-being mentor is a trusted person who will discuss your results and provide insights in areas you cannot see. They will also provide direction to help you grow. Ideally, this profile, when used well, will help you become healthier in all areas of life and better able to navigate your leadership responsibilities.

Access the assessment here https://vervelead.com/tools/#profile

Let's now look at the Core Competencies (Vital Spirituality, Thriving Relationships, Emotional Intelligence, Sustainable Life and Reduced Risks) and their behavioural expressions. Even though you may recognize certain competencies as an area of strength, I encourage you to explore all of them and find someone trusted with whom you can have an honest conversation, following your initial tour of this profile. I will give more information on how to find a mentor in the next chapter.

Competency One: Vital Spirituality

Has an intimate relationship with God that is life-giving and life-changing.

Vital spirituality is the cornerstone of a healthy Christian leader because all other competencies depend on the spiritual health and relationship with Jesus. Healthy lifestyle, sustainable work and effective leadership all flow from a solid understanding of a person's own beliefs and principles. Living with vital spirituality means that the scriptures are relied on to provide guidance, that intentional time is made for God with prayer and reflection, and that the leader is aware of God's power and presence throughout the day. This relationship with God transforms a healthy Christian leader into the best versions of themselves. The behaviours associated with vital spirituality are:

1. Aligns identity in Christ with scripture.
2. Engages in a rich prayer life.
3. Experiences God's involvement in all areas of life.
4. Exhibits a transformative connection with God.

Competency Two: Thriving Relationships

Demonstrates thoughtful understanding of others, and intentionally develops and maintains close connections.

Healthy leaders have a strong support system behind them: people who love them, who can provide perspective and honesty, who want what is best for them. A healthy Christian leader tends to their relationships carefully, making an effort to give as much as they take, to listen actively, and intentionally change behaviour if they see that it is damaging to others. A healthy leader forms secure attachments to those around them and maintains necessary boundaries. A healthy leader is compassionate in relationships, helping them to work through conflict, to hear when they are wrong and to seek to grow stronger and healthier connections with their community. A healthy leader knows how to apologise as well as forgive.

1. Builds secure attachments.
2. Adapts to improve meaningful connection with others.
3. Communicates transparently, effectively, and wisely.
4. Manages conflict well.
5. Demonstrates forgiveness.

Competency Three: Emotional Intelligence

Understands and manages own thoughts and feelings to strengthen well-being.

Emotional intelligence is crucial in every area of life: working through conflict with co-workers, meeting new people, interacting with strangers, handling tension between old friends… there is no limit to the positive effects of this competency. Some people develop these skills from a very young age and are naturally adept at understanding and regulating their thoughts and feelings, and expressing them appropriately. Others struggle to learn these skills. However, we can grow and increase our emotional intelligence through making time to practise self-awareness and humility, by taking care of our emotional needs, and by listening to the word of God.

1. Grows in self-awareness.
2. Practises self-reflection.
3. Maintains emotional well-being.
4. Cultivates a Biblical mindset.
5. Self-regulates emotions.
6. Displays humility.

Competency Four: Sustainable Life

Takes actions and forms behaviours that enhance long-term viability.

A Christian leader may have other healthy competencies in spades, but without a sustainable life, the effectiveness of their skills will eventually diminish. No matter how wise, spiritual, well-meaning or hard working a leader is, well-being still should be a priority. A healthy Christian leader makes sure they are making time for processing, reflection and relaxation in their schedule, no matter how busy! Self-care can lead to feelings of guilt, as if one is acting selfishly or lazily, but everyone needs this time for themselves. Everyone deserves to feel rested and content, and good leaders know that without making some time to care for themselves, they can't effectively care for others.

1. Maintains self-control.
2. Manages stress.
3. Demonstrates personal responsibility.
4. Embraces necessary change.
5. Displays resilience.
6. Lives with purpose.

Competency Five: Reduced Risk

Assesses physical, emotional and spiritual vulnerabilities to minimise harm and maximise safety.

There are many threats and risks involved in being a Christian leader. It isn't just a job, it's a role that can drastically affect a community. It's not work one necessarily leaves at the door at the end of the day: there are deeper emotional strings, a spiritual calling and pressure from always being an example for others. A healthy Christian leader understands these risks and knows how to minimise them through creating margins and boundaries both for themselves and their community, caring for their well-being, and maintaining support systems and key relationships.

1. Responds to emergencies with readiness, calm and confident leadership.
2. Implements a plan for well-being.
3. Engages in accountable relationships.
4. Creates margins in life.

How to Best Use This Tool

The Health of a Christian Leader Assessment

To begin to understand the profile of the healthy Christian leader and the vision for health that accompanies it, we must begin with understanding ourselves. This can be the most difficult step because it requires an honesty and vulnerability that we don't often allow ourselves.

The Health of a Christian Leader Assessment will accelerate well-being transformation. Remember, the results are just a snapshot of where you are right now. They do not define your future; only offer some insight into the direction you might want to take to become a more effective leader. Here are some more questions to reflect on after you have taken the assessment, and always worth going back to as you continue your journey.

Post-Assessment Reflection

- What expectations did I have as I took the Health of a Christian Leader Assessment?
- How do I feel after assessing where I am now?
- What strengths/weaknesses surprised me?
- What is my first step?
- When will I plan for my next assessment and improvement process?
- Who and what can help me stay accountable?

As you walk the path of self-exploration, acting and making changes in your life, it is important that you consistently review your progress. I like to use after-action reviews. After-action review[1], or AAR, is a technique developed by the U.S. army to analyse an individual's progress. It helps to identify good and bad practices to make necessary changes. Formal AARs are still used by many organisations. I encourage all mentors to use an informal AAR to check up on their mentee's progress whenever they pass major milestones. Consistent reflection is key to tracking patterns, analysing changes being made and

---

[1] Here is a helpful article on AAR https://hbr.org/2023/01/a-better-approach-to-after-action-reviews

will help both the mentor and the mentee see improvement.

Stop, Challenge, Choose

Once you have identified patterns or habits that are subtracting from your well-being and efficiency as a leader use the Stop, Challenge, Choose technique[2]. This can help you take action, especially when discussed with another person. Adrienne, my wife, and I have both identified that for me eating, drinking too much and falling asleep while watching movies were patterns I displayed when I was burnt out. This led me to see some actions I could stop, actions I could challenge and what I could choose to do instead. In my case, drinking less, eating healthier and making sure I was getting enough sleep in bed were all small but effective ways to begin to make positive changes in my life.

As you explore the different competencies of a healthy leader and the behavioural expressions that accompany them, you'll be asking. 'What behaviours would I like to cease? What could I start doing instead?'

Mentoring Relationships

You will want to find a mentor who seeks to help you be everything that God wants you to be. A mentor should be a few steps ahead of

---

[2] Formulated by Dr Wayne Anderson https://www.habitsofhealth.com/product/stop-challengechoose/

you in life and understand your passions and your spirituality. A good mentor listens well and only gives direction when it is essential. They don't judge or manipulate. They are compassionate, confidential and trustworthy.

Scripture shows that God does not mean us to journey alone. The mentor/mentee relationship arises again and again. In the Old Testament, Elijah took Elisha as a disciple and protege, guiding and teaching him what he knew. When Elijah was taken up to heaven, he left Elisha to continue his work.

Likewise, in the New Testament, Jesus guided and taught his twelve disciples and others—his mentees—who continued his work. The Apostle Paul took a mentoring role with Timothy, choosing him as a potential great leader, someone who would listen well and face challenges head-on. Paul spoke like a father, calling Timothy to rise above timidity into courage, power and love. He began by teaching Timothy, then worked closely alongside him, and finally, Paul sent Timothy out on his own, trusting he was wise enough to begin to mentor others. *You have heard me teach things that have been confirmed by many reliable witnesses. Now teach these truths to other trustworthy people who will be able to pass them on to others.*

2 Timothy 2:2 (NLT)

The use of strong mentors is a recurring recommendation in my work, and something I have seen lead to great transformation again and again. We find incidental mentors throughout our lives, but I believe that an intentional mentor will take any Christian leader further in their transformative journey than they could ever possibly go alone or with incidental mentors. Finding a second perspective outside of your own, one that comes from someone with wisdom, empathy and experience, will allow you to see and understand so much more about yourself. A mentor can help you find the right action steps to take, to see a clear path ahead of you when you may not. They may offer honest insight that you don't necessarily want, but truly need to hear in order to grow.

The relationship between mentors and mentees is symbiotic. For mentors, it comes down to the principle of making disciples and passing on what we know/experience to others. We're not just designed to be the recipient of wisdom and guidance, but also to offer it. For mentees, we need mothers and fathers in the faith who can guide and develop us to be everything that God wants us to be. We need those who can recognize our undeveloped gifts and potential and call us forward to live up to our possibilities.

Ephesians 2:20 (NLT) says, *Together, we are his house, built on the foundation of the apostles and the prophets. And the cornerstone is Christ Jesus himself.* This house cannot survive or grow larger if we are not imparting what we have learned to the next generation. Discipleship and mentorship are ways to stand on the shoulders of giants, not to make carbon copies, of course, but to use new thoughts and skills to make something bigger and more beautiful than before.

To recap, look for these qualities in a potential mentor:

- seeks to help you be everything that God wants you to be
- is a few steps ahead of you in life
- understands your passions and your spirituality
- listens well and only gives direction when it is essential
- doesn't judge or manipulate
- is compassionate, confidential and trustworthy

If you are looking for an experienced mentor, check out the Verve Lead website: https://vervelead.com/mentoring/. We can help you find the mentor who is right for you.

A Window into Ourselves

Mentors help mentees to see parts of themselves that they might not see otherwise.

In psychology, there is a tool called the Johari window. It was created by psychologists Joseph Luft and Harrington Ingham in 1955[3] and is still used to explain the relationships we have with ourselves and with others. I have used the Johari window for many years to help explain the value of mentorship.

The Johari Window shows four quadrants of an individual: Open, Façade, Blindspot and Unknown.

Open: This is the area that is known both to us and to others. It is what we openly express, and how we consciously act around other people.

Facade: This is the area where we hide ourselves from others: where we conceal aspects of ourselves like embarrassing traits, secret desires or past traumas that we are not ready to share.

Blindspot: This is where our blind spots live: things those around us see, but of which we are not conscious—subconscious tics,

---

[3] https://static1.1.sqspcdn.com/static/f/1124858/28387950/1617395004320/THE+JOHARI+WINDOW.pdf

mannerisms or certain qualities.

Unknown: This area remains unknown to us and those around us. An example might be buried childhood trauma that the brain has selectively and subconsciously suppressed.

	Known to Self	Known to Others
Known to Others	Open	Blindspot
Not Known to Others	Façade	Unknown

Finding a mentor who can see us clearly is the most effective way to begin to understand the full self. We need someone to shed light on our blind spots: someone we can trust to be wise, honest and open. A mentor can help recognize things we are hiding from our conscious selves and can help us feel safe enough to explore other areas.

Finding a good mentor who is right for you specifically can be difficult and overwhelming. A lot of people don't know where to begin searching or what to look for when testing the water with potential mentors. Mentors themselves need to take time to talk to potential mentees, understand their goals and struggles before reflecting on whether it is the right fit.

Here are a few different types of mentoring relationships.

Informal Mentor This might look like meeting up for coffee with a respected friend or colleague to discuss struggles and goals. Often the nature of the relationship is implied, but there is no contract.

Formal Mentor This would be a relationship that is intentional and defined, with set times to meet and with the implicit goal of growing as a person or professional.

Professional Mentor This means working with a professionally trained mentor, whom you pay for their time and expertise.

All these relationships can be incredibly helpful to a leader, and each has its own pros and cons. Casual mentoring feels low-risk and can be flexible, not to mention usually being free. However, formal and professional mentors are often more prudent as they have experience and training, along with clear boundaries and contracts to keep both members safe.

Here are some tips to help you find the mentor that is right for you.

- Look into what other people say and think of your potential mentor, through word of mouth or professional reviews.
- Explore boundaries, expectations, needs, frequency and payment before committing.
- Avoid dual relationships like going to a family member, close friend or inline manager, which create blind spots and come with natural biases. It is best to work with someone who has some healthy distance from your personal and professional life.
- Consider the checklist below.

Mentor Checklist

- Does my mentor help me see what others see about me?
- Do they help me see what God only sees?
- Do they help me face what I hide from others?
- Do they aid transformation in my life?
- Do I feel fully seen and understood when discussing issues?
- Do they help me to feel ownership for changes in my life?
- Do they spend more time talking or listening/asking questions?
- Do they help me create action plans for growth as well as listening to my struggles?

COMPETENCY ONE

Vital Spirituality

Has an intimate relationship with God that is life-giving and life-changing.

Spirituality is the core of every Christian leader's perspective, values and beliefs. Spirituality will affect teaching, relationships, views and judgements of others and will influence a leader's work, home life, hopes and every action made. This is true even of secular leaders; the core philosophy of any person will shape the way they lead their community. If a leader has an unhealthy spirituality, if they are lacking vitality, that will pervade everything they do, creating an environment that feels false, hypocritical or empty. People who look to this leader will struggle with their own spirituality, potentially risking their well-being, especially if it is clear the leader is doing nothing to revitalise this core area. While everyone goes through moments of doubt and distance in faith, a healthy leader will communicate honestly, share their doubts, lean on their mentors, friends and family and use their shortcomings as an opportunity to learn and grow into a stronger, more vital person.

There are four behavioural expressions of Vital Spirituality in a healthy Christian leader:

1. Aligns identity in Christ with Scripture.
2. Engages in a rich prayer life.
3. Experiences God's involvement in all areas of life.
4. Exhibits a transformative connection with God.

In this chapter, we will take an in-depth look at the importance of Vital Spirituality, and how these behaviours affect us as leaders and people.

Behavioural Expression One:
Aligns Identity in Christ with Scripture

> **H** Shares energetically with others what God is saying and routinely implements His precepts from scriptures into one's personal identity and actions.
>
> **M** Senses God's voice occasionally when reading scriptures, which results in modest impact on one's personal identity and actions.
>
> **L** Practises religious rituals and reads scripture as duty, but finds it dull, with no sense of God's precepts from scriptures impacting one's personal identity and actions.

How is my Relationship with Christ?

Relationships that pour into our emotional tank are one key toward enduring health. However, when we are depleted, we don't have the energy to give to these relationships and we withdraw. This reduces the replenishment we get from them. Those of us who have experienced high emotional depletion know that our relationships, including our relationship with God, become strained and suffer.

Recent academic research, Duke University's <u>The Clergy Health Initiative</u> and the University of Notre Dame's <u>Flourishing in Ministry</u>, show a direct correlation between emotional well-being and the vitality of relationship with God.

While our human connections can falter without equal energy pouring into the relationship, Christ will always be present and never waver. God will be there for you when you are burnt out and understand when you are depleted. God brings freedom and new life to His people. He brings hope and joy. *A cheerful heart is good medicine, but a crushed spirit dries up the bones.* Proverbs 17:22 (NIV)

Remember, though, that our relationship with Christ grows and thrives when *we* take time to spend with Him—time which can replenish our spirits in a way that other relationships cannot. Time with Him builds vital spirituality.

Finding Replenishment Through Your Relationship with God

Let's look at one area—our reading of the Bible. Reading and reflecting on that reading will validate and strengthen your spiritual identity.

In the darkest days of burnout, I found it difficult to read. The physical and emotional state caused a loss of focus. My emotions were so numb, and nothing I read sunk in. I could not even engage in a church service. Looking back, I see that as I approached burnout, my reading became dull, and God's voice got quieter and quieter as emotional wax built in my spiritual ear.

For many years, I had read the Bible from cover to cover, eagerly devouring all I could. I can still remember the initial feeling of finding His voice in the pages as words leapt out and engaged my heart. So impactful was His voice that I couldn't wait to share what I read with others. It gave me energy and strength.

In the pit of depression, I heard His voice saying, *The Lord is my shepherd, I will not want.* (Psalm 23). I wasn't sitting reading, but walking by my pool, when the words just bubbled up in my spirit. For three months, that is all I heard. Then, 'He lets me rest' was added. After about six months, I started reading again, and once again, I heard His voice in what I read.

During this time, I discovered that the picture I had of myself was so distorted compared to God's picture of me. I wanted to start seeing myself as God did.

So, I went back to this Bible verse:

See what great love the Father has lavished on us, that we should be called children of God! And that is what we are! The reason the world does not know us is that it did not know him. 1 John 3:1 (NIV)

At that point, I started to wonder, 'Who am I? What's my identity?'

I could see that there was a tremendous gap between what I was feeling and perceiving about myself and what God saw. In an attempt to bridge this gap, I read 1 John 3:1 every morning to affirm God's picture of me. Gradually, I understood that my identity in God isn't based on the amount of time that I spend reading or praying. Rather, it's based on what God has done for me.

In difficult times, His Holy Spirit will remind us of verses that will water our soul.

Sometimes, we may be so physically sick that we cannot feed ourselves and must regain health and strength to be able to do so. Similarly, we need to be well enough to be able to read scripture to feed ourselves spiritually.

If it's difficult to read, go for a walk, sit for a moment, ask this question, 'What's one thing I know God says about me from the scriptures?' Look for a verse that is positive and affirms your identity. Write that down and read it. Let it sink in and speak to who you are. Over a couple of months, add to the list. Let these become a soundtrack for you, affirming and strengthening your identity in Christ.

One simple thing that can help is to change the version of Scripture that you read. This can add new life and colour. Finding an accompanying guide or book to provide questions for reflections can also add much to your experience. Another very powerful aid is to join a small group where the scriptures are shared. Other people's revelations can spark a revelation in you.

My prayer for you is that you not only hear God's voice while reading the scriptures but that you implement these words in your own life. I pray His voice energises you to share your passion with others.

Healing Derives From Acceptance

Starting with that single verse helped to reform and reshape who I am. Later, I added five more Bible verses that speak about my identity in Christ. I came to a place of healing based on acceptance of my God-given identity. There was no sense of having to perform. However, out of gratitude, love and renewed energy, I could once again share God's word with others.

The health of your relationship with God is reflected in your emotional health. Upon understanding the image God has of you, you will gain the self-confidence and affirmation you deserve as a child of God.

Look again at the alignments of this behavioural expression. Where do you see yourself after reading this section?

Reflection Questions

- Which Bible verses speak to me about who I am in Christ?
- Is there a gap between God's plan for my life and my own plan?
- Am I confident and content with the identity I create, or the one God has bestowed upon me?
- What voices are shaping my identity?
- What can I do to build my identity with Christ?
- What behaviours do I need to cease?
- What can I start doing instead?

Behavioural Expression Two:
Engages in a Rich Prayer Life

> **H**   Talks with God unceasingly regardless of life circumstances and looks for opportunities to similarly pray with others.
>
> **M**   Talks with God regularly and occasionally prays with others.
>
> **L**   Prays infrequently.

Healthy Prayer Life is a Benchmark of a Christian Leader

During my burnout, I had a difficult time praying. I shifted from presence, peace and life to striving and fighting in my prayers. My words became harder and angrier, strident and aggressive. My prayer time reflected my perception that life was hard going. The adrenaline that was fuelling me invaded my prayer life making it difficult to focus and connect with Jesus. I was also losing the desire to pray with others. Adrenaline is designed to be a friend to help us through crises, but consistent adrenaline begins to wear away at life.

My prayer life before burnout was like Adrienne's childhood memory of cooking a crayfish (Australian rock lobster). Not having experience, her parents placed the live cray in hot water. Immediately, its ten legs sprung to action to climb out of the pot, causing a great commotion. Likewise, when I was in hot water I would pray. Prayer was a lifeline.

Anxiety and worries lifted, and peace came. I prayed not only in trouble but also in good times. Jesus is my friend, and I normally started my day talking to him. It was intimate and connected.

The advice of the day was to put the cray in room temperature saltwater and turn on the heat. The cray would swim around, die quietly, turning crimson and ready to eat.

Similarly, the compounding heat of stress gradually depleted my emotional well-being. The emotional depletion was killing me spiritually. I kept swimming not realising I was spiritually dying. Prayer became something I did out of habit and duty, but I felt that I had lost the relationship I once had with God.

Many Christians, even leaders in ministry, go through periods where they find prayer to be a chore, or something that feels empty and disconnected. Yet, prayer is essential to our health. Jesus when suffering intensely in the Garden of Gethsemane, took the disciples with him and encouraged them to pray:

Keep alert and pray that you'll be spared from this time of testing. For your spirit is eager enough, but your humanity is feeble. Mark 14:38 (TPT)

Jesus felt a need for them to join Him in prayer. He knew that there is something encouraging, uplifting and affirming when we pray together. Faith grows when we pray together. We all know the word 'amen'. It's a phrase which means 'I agree', 'Make it so'. How can you get an 'amen' when you are praying by yourself? When you get together with others and pray, there's a spiritual intimacy that happens, a connection that is built.

But what does a healthy prayer life look like? It's talking with God privately *and* looking for opportunities to pray with others. It's like having a deep friendship with someone: you have moments where you can talk with a continued flow of conversation, and there may be times of easy silence, calm moments of connection.

Recover Your Prayer Life

However, there can be challenges when praying.

When prayer has an intensity that derives from perceived lack, it's like a striving for something that is non-existent, and makes one feel bad about who they are. However, if prayer starts with a contentment in who we are in Christ, then no matter what the storm, prayer will triumph every time. Alive and vital prayer feels like a bubbling deep within.

When a relationship with God is poor, we find ourselves praying infrequently and becoming distanced from Him. This may be because we're feeling flat emotionally, that we have nothing to offer. In the early stages of burnout, I found I couldn't engage in prayer like I could previously. I had to rest and repair before I started to hear God's voice once more and was able to talk with Him again.

Sometimes, it goes deeper than feeling flat or dejected. Long periods of silence between yourself and God can be an indicator that something else is going on in your heart. If you're feeling empty, reach out. Talking to someone can help you to understand that the situation can get better. Whether you've been hurt by a trusted friend, or your life hasn't ended up how you had hoped it would, or you deliberately turned your back on God and have done something you know you shouldn't have: you can come back from any of these places. If it's the relationship that's suffering, then who can help you fix it? Relationships can be restored and that includes your relationship with God. He wants a close connection with you. Always.

It's important to note that if you are spiritually depleted, you are likely to be emotionally depleted as well. You may not be able to read the Bible or pray or even be aware of your spiritual needs because you are burnt out overall. If this is the case, you may need to rest and restore yourself. Once you are feeling replenished, find a trusted person who can help you restore your relationship with God.

Prayer with Others

It is also helpful to pray with others. It can remind you of the intimacy and the love within prayer: others' vitality spills into your own prayers. God encourages us to pray together as prayer shared with a group is a powerful message to both the Lord and to ourselves, allowing us to feel part of a community, and closer to those around us and God. Praying by yourself is clearly still good and meaningful, but it is something very special when shared with others.

Make Time and Space for Prayer

We all have our own routines and preferences when we pray, especially on our own. One person may prefer to find a quiet room in their own home, while another may communicate best with God while walking in nature. Some like to pray first thing in the morning, others prefer the evening. One person might like silence, and another might like soft music. I like sitting by the pool in the early morning. I like to read a few of my favourite scriptures, take some deep breaths and pray.

While there are different ways to pray, there are a few things that seem to be true for all: to be uninterrupted, to be somewhere peaceful and without distractions. If you do not already have a place to go, it's time to find your place.

It's also important to make sure you are praying consistently and making it a part of your schedule. Plan and make the time if necessary. Everyone feels too busy at times, but slowing down and making time for God will always be worth it: you will feel more in control and less anxious afterwards.

Look again at the alignments of this behavioural expression. Where do you see yourself after reading this section?

Reflection Questions

- What would help me engage in a richer prayer life?
- What would help me to want to pray more with others?
- What about on my own?
- Is something preventing me from talking more with Jesus?
- Which of my behaviours are working against a rich prayer life?
- What can I stop doing in order to help my prayer life? (e.g. running on adrenaline)
- Does my energy level affect my prayer life?
- What behaviours do I need to cease?
- What can I start doing instead?

Behavioural Expression Three:
Experiences God's Involvement in all Areas of Life

> **H** Confidently shares past and present experiences of God's involvement in one's thoughts, conversations, and events.
>
> **M** Identifies personal encounters and experiences of God but struggles to recognise God's present involvement in one's thoughts, conversations, and events.
>
> **L** Has limited or no sense of God's involvement in one's personal life.

Where is God in Your Life? Cultivating a High Awareness of God's Interaction with Daily Life

Given the nature of the components of burnout—high depletion, high detachment and low satisfaction—it is little surprise that connection with God and awareness of His presence is also highly impacted. I write to tell you that even if you feel distance, He will still hang onto you. Matthew 28:20 (NIV) says, *And surely I am with you always, to the very end of the age.*

I had such trouble sensing God in my life during burnout. The numbness and the feeling of disconnection from God made it difficult to experience his presence. If you had asked me to say where I had seen God at work, the list would have been short and not recent. It was as if He used to be in my life, but now it was difficult to feel His presence.

As I rested in recovery, I began to see God's presence with me again. I am especially grateful for the key relationships of family and friends that endured through that difficult and dark time; through them, I could identify where God was working in my life. I finally recognised that I was loved by God during my burnout experience and that He was consistently present.

Then, as my connection with God grew again, I consequently saw a growth in my connections with people.

When you are low, it is easy to allow your mind to run away with negative thoughts and to be consumed by a lack of hope. It takes some discipline to make the shift from focusing on your weariness and loneliness to becoming aware and appreciative of where you see God working. When you are thriving, it is easier to sense God's involvement in all facets of life.

Where is God at Work? Who Can Help You See?

My mentor would ask me, 'How is your relationship with God? Tell me about what is happening?' He wasn't looking for frequency or time spent in prayer but rather how vital and real it was. He helped me see God's presence and His intervention in conversations, thoughts and life outcomes. Mentoring builds reflection ability. Where has God been at work in your life? Where is He at work? Can you note any times in the week when you experience God's intervention in conversations, thoughts and outcomes?

Each week, I review the past week's engagements and activities, asking, 'Where did I experience the presence of God?' This helps me build the muscle of reflection. I prepare a note in my reflections folder, Monday to Sunday, entering known appointments and responsibilities. When the week is done, I spend time reflecting. I created a template in Evernote, with the following questions:

- Where did I experience the presence of God?
- Where was it hard going?
- How is my emotional tank?
- Where was I critical or withdrawn in conversations?
- What behaviours do I need to cease?
- What can I start doing instead?

Creating a Vision of Health

There is also an incredibly helpful Examen from St. Ignatius that I like to practise every week, although it can be done as often as daily and as infrequently as each month:

1. Become aware of God's presence.
2. Review the day with gratitude.
3. Pay attention to your emotions.
4. Choose one feature of the day and pray from it.
5. Look toward tomorrow.

Look again at the alignments of this behavioural expression. Where do you see yourself after reading this section?

Behavioural Expression Four:
Exhibits a Transformative Connection with God

H Maintains an intimate relationship with God, resulting in continual spiritual and personal growth.

M Knows God personally, but without close intimacy, resulting in stagnation of spiritual and personal growth.

L Stays feeling disconnected from God. May be failing to resist personal temptations.

Building a Strong Foundation with God

What is your relationship with God built upon? I've found that for many Christians, there is often a feeling of guilt and obligation hammered deep into the bedrock of their relationship. Building based on feeling obligated may get you started, but if it is the sole motivator, then it's not sustainable for a healthy lifestyle. Religious duty can bring a sense of dullness when speaking with God and doesn't positively impact your personal identity or change your behaviour. Obligation, guilt or shame won't bring you closer to God. For instance, do you read your Bible out of a sense of duty, obligation, or guilt? Does this bring you closer to God? Or do you read because you want to spend time in God's presence, to hear His voice, to know Him more?

During times like this, I hope you will ask yourself, 'What has caused this relationship to be dull and dry? Who am I in Christ? What is my spiritual identity?' In other words, build upon the solid foundation of your identity in Christ.

Allowing yourself to be honest about these emotions is the first step. God wants us to be honest and transparent with Him and with ourselves. This will help build intimacy and trust, forming a solid foundation in your relationship.

Developing a Vital Connection with God

What do you do if reading the scripture is dull and you can't sense God's voice? This question is not uncommon in a Christian's spiritual journey: sometimes, we can just get in a rut doing the same thing over and over. Eventually, we'll sense a misalignment in what we consider our ideals and our current behaviours and feelings towards our faith. That's when we need to mix it up by doing something different. Make it fun again! This may look like switching to other books that will help you cultivate your spirituality, having a daily Scripture reading plan or installing a Bible app that delivers a scripture of the day in your inbox.

I know two other practical ways that can help you hear God's voice when it seems dull. One is being around people who have an obviously exciting, joyful and vital connection with God. The second is to chat with someone who is new in their faith, who radiates the vibrancy and gratitude of being given the amazing gift of salvation. Both kinds of people will spark your love for God and ignite again your vital connection with Him.

Other ways to help you hear God's voice may be to read the verses that you highlighted in your Bible through the years, notes you made in the margins and your entries in a God journal, and recall what was happening in your life at that time. Reflect on what God said to you then and how it made you feel about Him. You'll find that you will experience the same emotions and a closeness to God like you experienced in the past.

I encourage you to read verses that positively impact your spiritual journey, just as this Bible verse did for me:

> *Stop imitating the ideals and opinions of the culture around you but be inwardly transformed by the Holy Spirit through a total reformation of how you think. This will empower you to discern God's will as you live a beautiful life, satisfying and perfect in his eyes.* Romans 12:2 (TPT)

Strengthening a relationship is a lot like strengthening muscles. It requires a process of growth, deliberate focus and discipline. It begins with asking yourself, 'What do I want?' and 'What am I experiencing?' We need to understand where we are to move towards where we want to be, and how we can use our difficulties and pain to grow. In this case, we need to understand what our ideals and values truly are, to see how they shape our identity, and to know whether they are in line with our spiritual identity and God's plan for us.

So, ask yourself, 'What trials and difficulties are helping me to strengthen my 'muscles' in a relationship? Who is helping me?'

Do you have a spiritual mentor, like athletes have physical coaches?

God wants the connection, but it's up to you to make it happen. Being transformed in Christ and altering your mindset will empower you to live a beautiful life knowing that God says you are loved. This is your gift from the Father.

Reflection Questions

- How do I describe my current relationship with God?
- When was the last time I felt God speak with me?
- How did that affect me?
- Is my scripture reading based on religious ritual or duty?
- What behaviours do I need to cease?

- What can I start doing instead?
- Look again at the alignments of this behavioural expression. Where do you see yourself after reading this section?

COMPETENCY TWO

Thriving Relationships

Demonstrates thoughtful understanding of others, and intentionally develops and maintains close connections.

As for anyone, Christian leaders cannot be healthy on their own. No matter how self-reflective, how empathetic, how mature we are, we will have blind spots. Our own flaws and strengths are often clearer to those around us, especially those with whom we are closest, those we trust, and those who know our habits, our principles and our background. Part of being a leader is understanding when we need support, honesty and love, and when we need to reciprocate these to others. Understanding how to sustain healthy, secure relationships and how to handle conflict and communicate well are essential.

There are five behavioural expressions for Thriving Relationships:

1. Builds secure attachments.
2. Adapts to improve meaningful connection with others.
3. Communicates transparently, effectively, and wisely.
4. Manages conflict well.
5. Demonstrates forgiveness.

Behavioural Expression One:
Builds Secure Attachments

H Promotes a deep sense of contentment and belonging in relationships.

M Connects well, but may allow insecurities to cause either some detachment or need for control in relationships.

L Perpetuates either high detachment or toxic dependence in relationships.

Building Healthy Key Connections: Constructing Lasting Relationships

Healthy key connections are essential for emotional well-being. This is true for all people of influence irrespective of leadership title. Mums and dads, friends and colleagues are people of influence, as are teachers, coaches, pastors, supervisors and many more. Attempting to lead without enduring relationships can be done but is not sustainable.

We are designed by God to be in relationships: to see others and feel seen by them, to understand and be understood, to strengthen and encourage one another.

Healthy Relationships Endure Through Time and Difficulties

That's one of the special things about great parenting relationships.

Parents have seen us at our worst—nappies, tantrums, sickness, selfishness, teenage years—yet most often the relationship endures. Parents speak love, encouragement and blessings. They call out strengths and possibilities. Peace and safety flow through a parent's voice and embrace to even an adult child. A parent's presence brings all the words and affirmations of the past into the present moment. The flexibility of the relationships gives space for individual growth (children leave home) and yet deep connection endures.

The Problem of Emotional Landfill

Emotional health affects relationships. Being unwell emotionally puts pressure on relationships; people grow distant, become irritable, over-indulge in bad habits. It can be an uncomfortable realisation for many that they could be the problem.

It has become culturally acceptable in our disposable world to discard relationships. With the high focus on self, if a person is not getting what they need or want, they can simply seek it out elsewhere. Just as disposing of plastics causes a landfill problem, disposing of relationships causes an emotional landfill problem. The breakdown in relationships leaves a residue in our emotions which affects the healthy flexibility needed.

One effect is a fear of rejection which may make a person hold back and not connect, or act either with over-flexibility or inflexibility.

On one hand, rejection can make people become overly flexible, allowing themselves to be taken advantage of, as they try to not get hurt again.

On the other hand, rejection can make people become inflexible in relationships, becoming manipulative, controlling and abusive, as they try to guard against loss.

It can be a difficult tightrope to walk.

Insecurities make people withdraw in relationships. They stop people from giving a word of encouragement, cause them to second-guess themselves and overthink what they were going to say. Insecurities take the focus away from the other person and move it to self. 'Will they still like me if I say this?'

An emotionally unwell person will withdraw, showing their detachment in blindness to connection bids—those little comments of, 'What are you doing later?', 'Let's catch up', 'I'm going to the beach on Saturday', followed by a pause that implies, 'Would you like to come?' A trail of broken relationships is an indicator that a person is not emotionally well.

We need healthy connections to thrive. Encouragement pours strength into our well-being. Healthy leaders go out of their way to strengthen and encourage, so take some time to think, 'Who can I encourage today?' Let's deliberately encourage and build strong connections.

Reflection Questions

- What connection bids have I missed this week?
- Who is not responding to my connection bids?
- Do I have an emotional landfill? Who could help me remove it?
- What behaviours do I need to cease?
- What can I start doing instead?

Behavioural Expression Two:
Adapts to Improve Meaningful Connection with Others

H Exhibits flexibility, while affirming deep, accountable connections during changing circumstances.

M Endeavours to live in harmony with others, but too easily avoids efforts to resolve difficult problems with interpersonal relationships.

L Exacerbates interpersonal problems with people through personal rigidity or provocation.

Adaptability: A Key to Thriving Relationships

Why do some relationships survive life's traumas, and some do not? The death of a child, major injury, acute sickness or intense financial pressure are some of the reasons given for relationship breakdown. Yet, some relationships grow stronger and deeper through similar difficulties. How do we support one another through our more difficult times of life?

One major characteristic of relationships that thrive in difficulty is their ability to adapt to the changes in circumstances. The flexible structure of their relationships helps them to endure.

Underlying this adaptability is the passion to live in harmony, conducting relationships like a musician making music with others, playing in the same key and cadence (structure), improvising to complement the other instruments' sounds (flexibility).

Think for a moment about the storms you have been through. Where have you had to be flexible in a relationship?

Chaos or Rigidity in Relationships

Chaos—people behaving unpredictably and acting on impulse—is the result of structural breakdown in relationships which may be caused by several things, for instance, sickness, unemployment, financial loss.

Rigidity can also be a result of a structural breakdown in relationships, but on the other hand, this is seen in the loss of flexibility. In this situation, the person finds solace in rigid structure and rules, and refuses to change or abandon this structure.

Abuse in its various forms also brings chaos or rigidity, and damages the ability to trust. When this is damaged, we need someone to help repair our trust. The good news is we can be healed.

Do you find changing circumstances in relationships difficult? Are you feeling controlled or manipulated? Do people in your world describe themselves as being neglected? If you answer yes, please chat with someone qualified to help you explore this further.

Understanding Your Attachment Style

We have learned how to relate from those who have related to us. For instance, our family of origin is strongly formative in our relationship behaviour. Secure attachments show us how to make secure attachments. Avoidant, fearful or anxious attachment styles likewise embed those styles in us. The first step in resetting the way we handle relationships, is to recognise our attachment style and whether it is healthy or not. Most psychologists recognize four major types of attachment styles: Secure, Anxious, Avoidant or Disorganized.

Secure: Healthy attachment based on trust and love. Can balance independence and intimacy in relationships.

Anxious: Seeks intimacy to the point of dependency, can be clinging and demanding in relationships. Deeply fears abandonment.

Avoidant: Independent and self-sufficient, in order to avoid intimacy. Has trouble forming or maintaining close relationships.

Disorganised: Both craves and fears intimacy, and reacts unpredictably when denied or given affection.

We should all be seeking to form secure attachments, but many of us struggle with how to make this happen. Our past relationships, beginning with our parents, teach us different ways to react to intimacy, and unfortunately, we often learn the wrong lesson. The good news is that we can grow and change. Pursuing God has helped me here. He does not avoid, fear or get anxious. He securely holds on to us. His love removes fear, and we can bring our anxieties to Him.

> *'Cast all your anxiety on him because he cares for you.'*
> 1 Peter 5:7 NIV

To learn more about attachment styles visit:
https://www.attachmentproject.com/blog/four-attachment-styles/

Investing Intentionally in Relationships

Intentional investment is like practising piano playing. It is the regular, deliberate discipline of sowing into the relationships that matter most, while giving space for each other's growth and development.

It's like parenting in a way; relationships go through stages, and sometimes, especially in the beginning, a relationship needs more attention. You have to be extra careful what you are putting into a new relationship; you want to say the right things in order to build trust and promote honesty. As the relationship grows and matures, this will happen more naturally, and both sides of the relationship can be more open with their feelings and opinions because trust and care has been established.

Most relationships go through phases of difficulty as well, moments of miscommunication, uncertainty, hurt and distrust, but through these stages, a healthy, secure relationship can endure and deepen.

Reflection Questions

- Am I more chaotic or rigid in my relationships?
- How do I adapt to change in relationships?
- What is my attachment style?
- How have I seen my attachment style affect my relationships?
- What steps can I take to help my current relationships thrive?

Behavioural Expression Three:
Communicates Transparently, Effectively and Wisely

> **H** Builds trust through active and compassionate listening, articulating clearly, and showing vulnerability.
>
> **M** Facilitates free-flowing communication, but allows fear of rejection to cause limited transparency.
>
> **L** Focuses and redirects conversations constantly to oneself or resorts to silence when one's voice needs to be heard.

Building Trust Through Listening and Affirmation

Have you noticed that when you talk with emotionally healthy influencers and leaders you feel listened to, affirmed and encouraged? Conversation with emotionally healthy people is easy and free-flowing. There is something about the way they consistently listen with empathy and speak with clarity that builds trust, making you feel valued, safe and belonging. There are no surprises—the relationship is dependable. Their transparent vulnerability gives you the sense that their world is not complete without their connection with you and that you can add value to them and their life.

Trust Impeders: Limited Transparency & Cynicism

If a fear of rejection underlies interactions, there will be limited transparency and we will cause a divide in the relationship. I wondered why at times people would say to me, 'I don't know what you are thinking,' or 'It would be really helpful for you to say some more.' Now I understand that my limited disclosure was due to a fear of rejection. I am so appreciative of my mentor who helped me be free from this fear.

One early change I noticed as I approached burnout was in the way I related and responded to others. I became more cynical and critical in attitude when expressing my intolerance of others' perceived ineptness. This concerned me as I was usually gracious in conversation. But I had become blunt and harsh. I am sorry for this. What was inside was flowing out. After dedicating myself to my own recovery and with the help and love from many people in my life, my graciousness was restored.

Two Symptoms of Emotional Sickness that Destroy Communication

LOSING YOUR VOICE

Well people communicate to connect, but sick people will often fall silent. In the same way that losing your voice is a sign of a sore throat, losing your voice in connections is a sign that something is not well. If someone has gone silent on you, don't take it personally, but journey with them to see them well. I am deeply appreciative of those who walked with me when I was sick.

We need the voice of those we love. Continued silence will cause people to look for some other voice. Dads, let your voice be heard. Mums, let your voice be heard. Lovers, let your lover hear your voice. Many times, I hear the reason for relationship breakdown as, 'He wouldn't talk to me.' Affairs often start this way.

LOSING SIGHT OF OTHERS

When people are emotionally unwell they easily lose sight of others. One sign of this is constantly bringing the conversation back to themselves, blocking free-flowing conversation by following a story with phrases like, 'This happened to me... ' and launching into a story about themselves. They see the other person's communication as an opportunity to tell something about their world.

The low measure of well-being makes them unable to build the relationship by asking questions like, 'What happened then?' or 'How do you feel about that?' or 'Tell me more.' They subconsciously need to endorse/promote themselves by telling their own story. Yes, there is a time and place for that. However, if it's a constant response to everything that is said by the other person, it quickly causes a chasm.

Reflection Questions

- Who am I most transparent with?
- Where can I increase vulnerability and transparency?
- Am I afraid to speak up? Do I avoid certain topics? Do I evade the truth when uncomfortable?
- Have I lost sight of those who matter?
- What behaviours do I need to cease?
- What can I start doing instead?

Behavioural Expression Four:
Manages Conflict Well

H Seeks understanding of critical issues without attacking persons, and assertively seeks resolution without aggression.

M Shows courage to resolve misunderstandings, but tends to personalise rather than objectify critical issues. Does not usually express one's own needs or feelings.

L Avoids conflict whenever possible and capitulates to its consequences. May become emotionally volatile when confronted about critical issues.

Two Steps to Managing Conflict

A young man I didn't know called. He needed some help. He had become very angry with a member of his extended family and was, understandably, boiling. He perceived he had done his best and was being unjustly treated.

'What do I do?' he asked.

My advice was, 'Take a breath, go for a walk, get calm and then go and talk with them.'

He texted back that evening, 'All is resolved. Thank you for your help.'

Regulate Your Own Emotions

The first step to prepare for confrontation is to regulate your own emotions. Your emotions influence others. Emotions rub off—they are transferred, caught like a virus. If this young man had gone to sort out the difficulty while angry, his anger would have spilled over, and things would have gotten loud, more strained and probably not ended with reconciliation.

To regulate emotions, give yourself some space to let them settle, try counting to ten, removing yourself, or taking a walk if you have the time. This could help you understand the overall situation and control your emotions, so they don't hijack the outcome.

Confront the Issue not the Person

The second step that emotionally healthy leaders and people take is to confront without capitulating. Of course, if you are in the wrong, please acknowledge, accept responsibility and seek forgiveness. There are times when wisdom says to let it go.

However, confrontation is a necessary part of healthy relationships. Healthy leaders carefully articulate their concerns having wisely set the time and place. They are able to express 'I need' and 'I feel' and work to resolve. It takes healthy emotional well-being to be assertive like this.

Courage is required to address and resolve conflict because the outcome is unpredictable. Some do not handle conflict well because they are prone to becoming defensive, some tend to shut down emotionally and some retaliate with anger.

Confrontation is like the discipline of children, which is not about inflicting punishment but about bringing change that enhances relationships.

Two Steps to Expressing Your Needs and Feelings

I used to avoid conflict. This was so unhelpful as a leader of a church. In fact, it was unhelpful for any relationship or leadership role. My stance was rationalised by thinking that not confronting is more loving. But it is not. Genuine care calls people to change even when this call may not be received well.

I'd not learned to confront effectively. Early on, I experienced some people who when confronted would explode. In thinking this was normal, I refrained from confrontation, not wanting them to emotionally vomit on me.

Now I see that they were emotionally unwell.

Don't Take It Personally

It took me some reorientation (regarding the personal-or-not nature of conflict) to realise that confrontation to resolve difficulties is a key to building connections.

As a lead pastor, I couldn't avoid confrontation completely. Sometimes people got disgruntled, and in announcing their departure, would come with their complaints. I took the confrontation personally and I clammed up, not expressing my own needs or feelings. After all, they were rejecting me and blaming me for their unhappiness.

In the journey from burnout to health, my mentors helped me develop self-confidence and self-value. I rebuilt robustness and resilience. I gained strength to learn to confront. One important step was to develop assertiveness and so be able to express what I feel and need.

Don't Make It Personal

Another key step is to not make your confrontation personal. It's like parenting where you call out the behaviour not the person. You don't say, 'You are a bad boy for hitting your sister.' You say, 'Hitting your sister is wrong. We don't do that. Here is your consequence.' God always loves the sinner, but not the sin. We should do likewise.

Healthy leaders engage in healthy confrontation to build enduring, robust relationships.

Reflection Questions

- Do I avoid conflict?
- Do I take conflict personally?
- What behaviours do I need to cease?
- What can I start doing instead?

Behavioural Expression Five:
Demonstrates Forgiveness

> **H** Releases others graciously from their wrongdoings.
>
> **M** Maintains some grudges when feeling justified.
>
> **L** Recounts others' wrongs readily, and cuts offenders from key relationships. May make excuses for bad behaviour or struggle with resentment, anger or revenge.

The Power of Sorry

During the process of recovery, I came to the realisation that burnout didn't just affect me, but that others connected to me were also impacted. This realisation was quite confronting. When pain is intense, we often lose sight of what is happening in other people because typically we are focused on ourselves.

Burnout by nature has three components or indicators—high depletion of the emotional tank, high disengagement in key relationships, and low satisfaction with work/accomplishments. All the components of burnout put pressure on key relationships. When our tank is empty we have nothing to give, so we disconnect from relationships. Low satisfaction with work makes us highly critical. The adage 'one suffers, all suffer' is true in this case. It took me some time to see this. As the realisation of the impact on others dawned, I saw that my sickness caused pain. Two emotions were strong in this realisation—gratitude for those who loved me through this time and helped my healing, and sorrow for the difficulty they and others experienced.

Making Apologies

What could I do about the impact on others? I decided on conversations with them. I set aside intentional time and made it clear that I was focusing on the person in front of me. We met in places with few distractions. I turned off my phone. I allowed people to talk freely. There I heard things I didn't always want, but needed to hear.

I also found that writing my feelings in letters was helpful mainly because I could carefully and thoughtfully express my sentiments. In my letters of thank you and apology, I attempted to express recognition of the difficulties others experienced and appreciation for them as people.

Making these apologies was difficult and required a lot of vulnerability and humility, but what happened after writing and sending these letters was wonderful, much better than anticipated or expected. I was surprised by the effect on me. Writing helped the healing and gave me clearer sight. It was also healing and freeing where relationships had been broken. Consequently, people expressed their appreciation and gratitude for my apology. I didn't expect to go back to the way our relationships were, because you can't, as life moves on. Letter writing may not be for everyone, but making the effort to speak your heart to the people in your life that you have hurt is such a powerful gesture. Saying sorry and the granting of forgiveness are standard operating procedures for healthy relationships to develop. The Bible says, *Love keeps no record of wrongs.* 1 Cor 13:5 (NIV)

Reflection Questions

- Do I need to send someone a letter of apology/thanks?
- What do I need to say?
- What behaviours do I need to cease?
- What can I start doing instead?

COMPETENCY THREE

Emotional Intelligence

Understands and manages own thoughts and feelings to strengthen well-being.

Behavioural Expression One:
Grows in Self-Awareness

> **H** Continually evaluates oneself honestly, despite seeing undesirable aspects of the self-picture.
>
> **M** Reacts to, rather than endeavours to understand, emotional and physical distress.
>
> **L** Fails to recognise or give space to emotions and related physical reactions.

Building Emotional and Physical Self-Awareness

Developing self-awareness is a major requirement for sustained emotional health. However, all of us have some awareness and some blindness of who we are.

Creating a Vision of Health

The Johari Window technique gives insight to this. Some areas of our life are visible to others and ourselves. We have a secret area where things are hidden from others. We have areas we can't see but others can see. And then there is the 'God-only-knows area', invisible to both others and us.

During long road trips when our children were young, we played the game, 'I can see something that you can't see, and it starts with...' A lot of fun and a great passer of time. It's amazing how awareness of your surroundings is built by playing this game. Similarly, through focus, you can build emotional and physical self-awareness. It's only as we build awareness that we begin to see our blindness.

Becoming aware of what is happening physically helps us to recognise the depth of what is happening emotionally. Physical reactions—for example, hands shaking under duress, dry mouth, or feeling fatigued—are helpful indicators if we pay attention to them.

During the time of recovery from burnout, with help from my mentor, I came to see that my practice was to give little space for recognising or processing emotions. I thought I was self-aware, but I was blind to myself. Just prior to my fortieth birthday, my younger sister (thirty-two years old) tragically died. Rosanne had given birth five days earlier to her third child.

Rosanne and I were very close. She was one of the young people who had decided to follow Jesus the first time I gave a public call for commitment—something that was so special to me. In our last conversation, she told me that they had called the new child Timothy—my middle name. I felt the loss of Rosanne deeply, yet hardly recognised or talked about it. Few people knew how I really was. I didn't take time off other than to attend the funeral.

We had planted a church two years previously and we were in go-mode. I didn't give myself space to grieve. I didn't know how. In hindsight, it would have been great to have a mentor to unpack the grief, and thereby, begin healing.

Years later my mentor helped me to see that blindness to emotions also leads to blindness to corresponding physical reactions. One common physical reaction to grief is weariness. My mother-in-law told us how six weeks after the passing of her husband, she found it very hard to get out of bed. There was nothing wrong physically, other than the body dealing with the recent loss. The adrenaline which helped her through the death/funeral and initial grieving had drained away leaving her feeling lethargic. Recognising that the physical reaction was normal was helpful in processing her grief.

Reflection Questions

- Have I discovered any blind spots in my life?
- Who helped me recognize these blind spots?
- Are there any physical signs that manifest when I am in stress? Could I use these as a sign to check in with myself emotionally?
- What behaviours do I need to cease?
- What can I start doing instead?

Behavioural Expression Two:
Practises Self-Reflection

> **H** Sets aside regular time for self-reflection and acts on constructive insights gained.
>
> **M** Increases in understanding of emotional blind spots and their physical effect but without acting accordingly.
>
> **L** Gives little to no time to the habit of self-reflection.

Self-Reflection is a Catalyst for Change

Self-reflection is a competency that many people avoid either intentionally or subconsciously. It can be scary to see our darker sides and after we understand ourselves, it means we have no excuse to avoid the difficult changes required to grow as a person.

Once, I believed self-reflection to be a dangerous practice leading to self-centeredness and selfishness. I was wrong. While it may worsen an existing inclination to be self-centred and selfish, it is not necessarily an entry point to either. To safeguard this, seek to grow in your awareness of God and others while you also practise awareness of self.

The three are interrelated. We are impoverished and diminished if our focus is only God and self. We are lost if our focus is merely ourselves and others.

When I exercise my self-reflection, I start with becoming aware of the presence of God and where He was with me during the week. Then I reflect on my actions, thoughts and behaviours in my key relationships.

What Does Self-Reflection Give Access to?

The key to open the door of self-reflection is practice. What's behind the door? Where does it take you? The practice of self-reflection builds self-awareness which then empowers you to act on gained insights.

Not only does self-reflection help you recognise your behaviours and emotions, but also to observe your thought patterns and their corresponding impact. In turn, this helps clarify who you want to be. Clarity in values and aspirations based on a realistic view of current behaviours, thoughts and emotions is a catalyst for change.

How Can I Begin to Practise Self-Reflection?

Like any other skill, self-reflection becomes most effective when it is practised at least weekly. For everyone, self-reflection will look a little bit different, but here is how I choose to do so:

As mentioned earlier, I have found this daily Examen practised by St. Ignatius to be a wonderful place to begin. I love the focus on the presence of God.

1. Become aware of God's presence.
2. Review the day with gratitude.
3. Pay attention to your emotions.
4. Choose one feature of the day and pray from it.
5. Look toward tomorrow.

On Mondays, I always reflect on my week overall. I have a template in an app (Evernote) and I label it for the coming Monday (e.g. Reflections 22nd April 2024). Then, I enter my appointments and schedules because I want to include them in the following week's reflections. If something significant and unexpected happens during the week, I open the note and make updates.

Here is my template I fill out every week:

- Reflections date
- Where did I experience the presence of God?
- Where was it hard going?
- How is my emotional tank?
- Any signs of burnout
  (e.g., Critical during conversation or withdrawn)

Who Can Help Me Understand My Self-Reflections More Clearly?

Sometimes, the emotions are big, and we need someone to help us unpack them and plot a path forward. A great mentor will help you self-reflect, give you feedback to help you see what you don't see and help you build ownership for change.

Self-reflection is a catalyst for change.

Reflection Questions

- Where did I experience the presence of God in the last week?
- When was it hard going?
- Am I experiencing any signs of burnout?
- Where was I critical of others?
- When was I withdrawn?
- What behaviours do I need to cease?
- What can I start doing instead?

Behavioural Expression Three:
Maintains Emotional Well-Being

> **H** Displays energy for life, love and work, and assists others in making changes in their lives.
>
> **M** Stays afloat during the normal challenges of life but falters in a crisis.
>
> **L** Stays in a state of emotional emptiness. May experience fatigue, numbness and ineffective decision-making.

Three Keys to Developing Emotional Well-Being

Healthy Christian leaders maintain emotional well-being. So how do we know we are well? How do we ensure our lifestyle is supporting sustainable well-being? Here are some tips.

1. Check your emotional tank

How are you emotionally? Are you feeling depressed, worn out or anxious? How are your relationships right now? What might be some factors that are contributing to your emotions and what could you do to restore your tank to full?

The key to maintaining your emotional well-being is firstly to take time to regularly reflect. This is wise. You should ask this question at least weekly: how full is my emotional tank?

You can also take our free Buoyancy Gauge here to help determine how you are emotionally: https://vervelead.com/buoyancy

2. Find a great mentor

Find a well-being mentor who can help you form a real picture of your emotional well-being.

Most of us, when asked how we are, will quickly respond without thinking, 'Great, thanks.' This cultural norm contributes to blindness in emotional well-being. A mentor will help you go further than the standard answer.

How can you ask the question of others and get a more realistic answer? For example, if you ask, 'What's been happening for you?' Or 'What's bringing you joy/pain at the moment?' and the mentee shrugs it off with a vague response, try a pause, leave a gap, and wait for a further comment. You know it's a good question to ask if they are pausing for several seconds; they are pondering it.

3. Intentionally charge your emotional energy

What helps you keep a phone supplied with power? Knowing that it needs charging. Checking the battery level and building in time for charging ensures that you have sufficient reserves. It's annoying to have a call end because they or you neglected to charge the phone. We can likewise crash if we aren't maintaining our emotional energy level.

If you are struggling with emotional energy, and how to recharge yourself, Verve Lead has many resources that can help you to see where you are struggling and how to address it: https://vervelead.com. You can also check out my previous book *Burnout and Beyond: The Danger of Depletion and the Path to Health*, which details my personal journey through burnout and recovering my emotional energy in the wake of this difficult time. You can buy my book on Amazon (paperback or Kindle versions).

Reflection Questions

- If my normal charge routine is not working, what changes can I make?
- Who can help me know how and when to charge my battery?
- What behaviours do I need to cease?
- What can I start doing instead?

Behavioural Expression Four:
Cultivates a Biblical Mindset

> **H** Filters attitudes and perspectives through scriptural principles rather than humanistic attitudes and perspectives.
>
> **M** Endeavours to filter attitudes and perspectives through scriptural principles, but allows negativity to cause self-doubt and indecision.
>
> **L** Anticipates and finds negativity constantly without filtering attitudes and perspectives through Godly principles.

Positive Thinking vs A Biblical Mindset

What does it mean to have a Biblical mindset? Many hear the term and think it means you read the Bible, attend church, be kind to others… normal Christian living. While this is correct, cultivating a Biblical mindset is much more. It means that we reframe our natural mindset through the scriptures, building an awareness and gratitude for God into our daily lives. It's more than a few acts, a few times a week. It's a lifestyle and a new way of thinking.

Much of a Biblical mindset is about limiting negative thought. So many people have a bad habit of anticipating the worst and adding stress to their lives; missed calls, texts and emails need to be read immediately in case they contain bad news. An important event is approaching and all they can do is play worst case scenarios out in their heads. They see someone on social media and immediately compare themselves to them, concluding that those people are happier, healthier, more talented and successful. The outcome of this comparison is that they don't want to engage because they have a poor self-picture. Confidence is undermined by negative thoughts: self-doubt and fear cause immobilisation.

A humanistic view would tell us that the opposite of negative thinking is positive thinking. Anticipate the good, live in the present, appreciate what is around you. That's all fine and true, but a Biblical mindset takes it further. It's more than positivity. It's finding peace within a deep trust of the Lord's divine plan.

The perspective that all things work together for good, and that God created us with only good in mind will be a deeper anchor than our emotions and simply thinking positively.

When I am struggling with negative thoughts, these are the verses I bring myself back to:

> *'For we are God's handiwork, created in Christ Jesus to do good works, which God prepared in advance for us to do.'*
> Ephesians 2:10 (NLT)
> *'And we know that God causes everything to work together for the*

> *good of those who love God and are called according to his purpose for them.'*
>
> Romans 8:28 (NLT)
>
> *'This is the day the LORD has made.*
> *We will rejoice and be glad in it.'*
>
> Psalm 118:24 (NLT)

This deep trust isn't based on circumstances but rather on the belief that God is at work in our lives and is always there for us. We are part of a grander story. We are valuable. We are loved.

Reflection Questions

- How can I stop anticipating bad news?
- Who can help me look for the good?
- Weekly reflection: Where is God at work?
- Daily reflection: Where have I seen blessings today?
- What behaviours do I need to cease?
- What can I start doing instead?

Behavioural Expression Five:
Self-Regulates Emotions

> H — Behaves responsibly toward oneself and others regardless of one's momentary feelings.
>
> M — Forgoes restraint when feeling uncertain or threatened.
>
> L — Reacts without restraint and regard to the impact of one's reactions on self and others.

Four Keys to Self-Regulate Emotions

It never feels good when people react without emotional restraint, especially with verbal abuse. I liken it to seeing someone throw up. However, this thoughtless reaction is often an indication that something deeper is going on with this person. As leaders, it is our responsibility to not respond negatively but to try to understand the true problem and help the person get well.

During my burnout, one of the signs that I was not emotionally well was that I became more critical in conversation. It became harder to hold my tongue, and cynical and critical words flowed. Kindness was replaced with a curt bluntness. I found it harder to act with restraint. The sicker I became, the less aware I was of how my actions hurt those around me.

Looking back at this time, I can't help comparing it to an angry moment I had in Grade 2. One very hot day, we were playing cricket at school. My mates saw I was not feeling good about my batting. They pushed and prodded me until I boiled in a rage. Reacting without restraint, I threw the bat, shouted angrily, chased, pushed, and punched. Eventually, I ran out of steam and recall feeling exhausted and very foolish. Even then, as a child, I recognized that this was an immature and inappropriate way to handle my feelings.

Here Are Some More Appropriate Ways to Respond

Delay your response. If it's an email, don't quickly fire an email back.

Withdraw if it's not safe. This gives you both time to cool down.

Set personal boundaries. What will you not tolerate in this conversation? What do you need to feel safe and respected? Often, it's helpful to share these boundaries up front, but there are times where it may not be necessary; you can hold yourself and those around you to these boundaries without making it a talking point.

Then, be assertive; express what you feel and what you need. Don't put up with the abuse.

Get someone else in the conversation. Show them your reply email or ask them to sit in on the meeting with you. Ask for help to word a response that does not stir up anger. Matthew 5:9 (NLT) reminds us, *'God blesses those who work for peace, for they will be called the children of God.'*

Take time to consider what is truth and what is emotion. Write down what you recall. Note what was said, and also, visible, measurable things, for instance, not that they were angry (that's your conclusion if they did not say they were angry) but that they were shouting, swearing, shaking, waving fists, red in the face... What accusation did they make? Ask yourself the question, why are they reacting this way? What is the underlying cause?

Reflection Questions

- Can I recall a moment I reacted strongly and without thought? How did it affect those around me?
- Are there any techniques that have worked for me in preventing inappropriate responses?
- Who can I ask to help me mediate a reactive situation?
- What behaviours do I need to cease?
- What can I start doing instead?

Behavioural Expression Six:
Displays Humility

> **H** Demonstrates a modest view of oneself as evidenced through altruism, empathy and curiosity to learn.
>
> **M** Displays appreciation of others' strengths and contributions but under pressure becomes closed-minded and thinks one knows best.
>
> **L** Tends to find solutions alone, perceives that one's own ability is superior, and resists constructive feedback.

Keys to Humility

When I was two, my parents took me on the train to Alice Springs in central Australia. My dad was an engine driver, so it was a special thing for me. During the journey, my mother gave me a tin full of biscuits for a snack. I looked around at all the people on the train and saw that they didn't have any biscuits, so I went around offering one to everyone on the train before I took a bite for myself.

Afterwards, I clearly remember my mother, who must have found this very endearing, telling me to 'never lose humility.' This stuck with me, that she considered this an act of humility, because I was putting others above myself.

What is Humility?

A common definition of humility is a modest or low view of one's own importance, humbleness. It is a lack of arrogance or self-interest. For me, it is closely connected with altruism; being able to value people and their needs even at the cost to you.

> *Don't be selfish; don't try to impress others. Be humble, thinking of others as better than yourselves. 4 Don't look out only for your own interests, but take an interest in others, too. 5 You must have the same attitude that Christ Jesus had. 6 Though he was God, he did not think of equality with God as something to cling to. 7 Instead, he gave up his divine privileges; he took the humble position of a slave and was born as a human being. When he appeared in human form, 8 he humbled himself in obedience to God and died a criminal's death on a cross.*
> Philippians 2:3-8 (NLT)

What Are Ways I Can Increase My Humility?

A key word here is curiosity. Curiosity about the people around us leads to understanding the strengths and skills of others, as well as what they have gone through to become the person they are now. The more understanding we have of a person, the more empathy we have for them. Empathy allows us to see others and ourselves with more clarity.

I once met with the lead pastor of a very successful mega church. He began by asking me, 'What are you good at, Don?' I thought for a minute and responded, 'I'm a great dad. My children are doing well and are following Jesus.' He then asked me if I had some messages on this that I could send to him. He said he wanted to learn how to be a great dad. His curiosity surprised me, and this demonstration of humility illustrated that you can learn something from anyone.

People who hang onto their wealth or position because it gives them a sense of self-importance can be destructive to those around them. Some amount of ambition is healthy, but letting it define who you are, or letting it get in the way of the well-being of others, makes for an unhealthy environment for yourself and everyone around you.

Hope for and work for the success of others. Several years back, we were appointed as Queensland State Directors for C3 and given the commission to mentor a young couple to be the future directors of Queensland. Since then, they have risen to be not only National Directors but also Global Executive Directors. A good leader should want to build others up to be everything they can be and do everything God calls them to. Develop others rather than keeping your position of importance by preventing the success of others. Desire that people around you to do as well as and better than you.

Show empathy. Showing that you value others through the sacrifice of time, finances, or effort can go a long way to remind you of your own humility. Everyone has bad days, or maybe even bad years. Seeing someone in a difficult situation and going out of our way to help, not only reminds us of where we've been but will make us grateful for where we are now.

Reflection Questions

- When do I display arrogance or selfishness?
- When do I display humility?
- Who can help me see myself more clearly and guide my next steps?
- What behaviours would I like to cease?
- What could I start doing instead?

COMPETENCY FOUR

Sustainable Life

Takes actions and forms behaviours that enhance long-term viability.

Behavioural Expression One:
Maintains Self-Control

- **H** Makes responsible choices based on sound judgement while keeping one's impulses under control.
- **M** Relinquishes sound judgement under pain or pressure, resulting in diminished disciplines.
- **L** Displays unsound judgement routinely through compulsive actions or impulsive choices.

Developing Self-Moderation

Everyone has something they just love: sweets, adrenaline, a cold beer... it's normal. When something is good, we want more, and occasionally, we overindulge. That's normal too. It's when we form real addictions that things get scary and serious. Dependency on a substance or experience can be very difficult to manage. Often, even a seemingly innocent thing can take a dark turn when a person becomes obsessed with it: shopping, watching TV, eating, going to the gym... Most of us just want to be able to enjoy these things on occasion, while avoiding building bad habits or reaching a state of dependency. So, we need to practise regulation and moderation.

Often, people have a prohibition attitude because they think others will judge them, or perhaps because of past negative experiences with a substance (e.g., an alcoholic parent). When you are a child this makes sense, but part of being a responsible adult is knowing how to set your own boundaries and moderate yourself. If we simply cut out everything we love, just because it could become a vice, we'd end up with a pretty joyless life and we'd lose the skill of moderation—a skill needed in many areas of life.

Adapting how you think about difficult or challenging experiences is the best way to handle your choices. Instead of making impulsive decisions, think ahead of how your choices will affect your day, how they will affect tomorrow. How will they affect your future in a year? If you can make smart decisions out of self-care instead of self-denial, the effects will last longer and feel better.

Growing the ability to say 'No' is a necessary skill when it comes to regulating. There is always a time to say 'No'. For instance, maybe it's when you are offered a drink the night before you have an early, important meeting, maybe it's after your second drink. It will depend on the situation, but learning how to gauge when you've had enough will allow you to still participate in things you love without regrets.

Here Are a Few Helpful Moderating Tips.

Know and understand your weaknesses and be familiar with what you tend to over-indulge in. Why this particular thing? Am I avoiding a feeling? Chasing a feeling? Searching for control? Understanding the root cause will help you understand the best way to control it.

Keep impulses under control. Setting limits, making boundaries and sticking to your plan will help make this easier for you.

Don't relinquish sound judgement under pressure. This can be a hard one when you are having a great time with friends or having a particularly stressful day. This is a time to ask what your future self would want you to do.

Set new targets and be encouraged. Don't shame yourself when you fail. Consider why this is so hard for you, set new goals and try again.

Break habits and have faith to step out of your comfort zone. It's never too late to make a healthy change for yourself. You don't have to be the life of the party, you don't have to be the one who finishes up someone's plate when they're done, you don't have to be the person posting multiple updates a week on social media. God wants you to take care of yourself, and if you put trust in him, and trust in yourself, you can make the changes you need.

Reflection Questions

- What are the vices that I over-indulge in?
- When do I tend to lose my moderation?
- What goals/boundaries/targets can I set to help me moderate my vices?
- Who can help me set these goals/boundaries/targets?
- What behaviours do I need to cease?
- What can I start doing instead?

Behavioural Expression Two:
Manages Stress

> **H** Develops awareness of stress and is proactive in mitigating its effects.
>
> **M** Shows an inability sometimes to set boundaries and allows unnecessary stress to accumulate.
>
> **L** Disregards stress level and over-exerts to the point of experiencing physical symptoms.

Managing Stress

Stress is a necessary part of life. Without it, we wouldn't grow. Work, relationships, personal goals—all these things naturally come with some amount of normal stress attached. The question is, how is the best way to handle it?

There are plenty of unhealthy ways: over-indulgence, avoidance, working non-stop... but how can we minimise and handle stress healthily? Two helpful ways are the ability to say 'no' and to engage help from others.

1. The Ability to Say 'No'

Saying 'No' is a skill. Most of us want to make the people around us happy. We want to be seen to be giving our all and working hard. So, whether we are saying 'Yes' to our boss's request for us to work late, or saying 'Yes' to meeting friends on an already busy evening when we are exhausted, it is often easier to say 'Yes' than ask for what we really need.

Saying 'No' when you are too stressed is different from just saying 'No' because you don't feel like it. There are times we must do things we don't feel like doing. Understanding the line between when you are pushing yourself and pushing yourself too much is the cornerstone of this skill set.

Reflection Questions

- Am I more stressed than I should be?
- What are my priorities this week?
- What tasks or obligations are outside my priorities?
- Can these be moved to another time?
- Have I made time to rest, relax and reflect this week?

2. Asking for Help

Our relationships are the best asset we have to mitigate stress. Having people we trust to talk to and process what we are going through, people that we can depend on when we feel lost, depressed or angry can keep us from falling off the edge and into burnout.

Often, we also need an outside perspective to be able to see our problems clearly. It can be hard to ask even our closest friends and family for help because of pride, fear of being an inconvenience, or discomfort with difficult conversations. However, no matter the reason, stress only builds and builds if we try to handle it alone.

Reflection Questions

- Who in my life can I turn to when I need help?
- What stops me from asking for help when I need it?
- How can I intentionally reach out to people around me when I need them?
- How can the people around me help me to gain clarity and perspective?
- What behaviours do I need to cease?
- What can I start doing instead?

Behavioural Expression Three:
Demonstrates Personal Responsibility

> **H** Takes ownership for the consequences of one's actions rather than blaming other people or circumstances.
>
> **M** Tends to self-isolate and problem solve alone when consultation with and support from others are warranted.
>
> **L** Takes no ownership for the consequences of one's actions and blames other people or circumstances.

Showing Agency and Taking Responsibility

Why We Need Agency

Agency is the capacity of individuals to act independently and to make their own free choices. Showing agency is a cornerstone of mature adults and implies taking responsibility for oneself.

We should all show agency in our finances, for example. To spend less than our income. Scott Pape in *The Barefoot Investor* details actions (beginning with taking responsibility for our financial decisions) to overcome a debt problem and become financially secure. Overspending is certainly a phenomenon of western culture and has become normalised. Often, we feel that we aren't getting paid enough, or everything around us is too expensive—true in some cases. However, the solution still begins with us taking responsibility and agency for how we spend our money.

Where Could I Show More Agency?

Agency isn't just about concrete things like money. During the eight months after I was diagnosed with burnout, I began to reflect on some things that I hadn't been able to see clearly when I was in the middle of my personal crisis. I realised that I played a part in the breaking of some relationships as I spiralled toward burnout. I had become withdrawn and critical, blaming people around me for anything that went wrong, and had no capacity for listening to what they had to say. I would simply think, 'That's just wrong' without asking any questions. Here's the big thing—I wasn't owning my part in conflicts.

If we display agency, we are taking responsibility for our choices rather than laying blame on others. Rather than leaving others to do what we should be doing, we are the ones who make things happen.

Reflection Questions

- How do I show agency? How could I show more?
- Where have I taken ownership of the consequences of my actions?
- Can I think of a time when I chose to blame someone for something that I actually had some responsibility for? Why was it so difficult to see my part in the problem?
- What behaviours do I need to cease?
- What can I start doing instead?

Behavioural Expression Four:
Embraces Necessary Change

> **H** Finds innovative solutions and makes changes when needed, even when changing is difficult.
>
> **M** Makes some constructive changes but often reactively rather than proactively.
>
> **L** Stays stuck in unproductive patterns, habits, and commitments.

What to Do in the Face of Change?

No matter who you are, or what kind of life you live, you will face change—good, bad and neutral. While certain changes in your life can be exciting (new job, getting married, having children) there is always something a little frightening accompanying change. Almost inevitably, change means you will lose one thing as you gain another. The more negative the change feels, the harder to process.

Some of us are quite adept at embracing change, while some of us try our best to avoid it. Think back to a time where you have attempted to avoid a change or dreaded an inevitable change. How did you feel before the change? How did you feel after it happened?

Sometimes, we even avoid good things out of fear because of the risk of being hurt or let down. Think about applying for your dream job or admitting feelings to someone you care about without the certainty that they feel the same way. It's scary and difficult, because of the fear of failure or pain. It often seems easier to avoid these situations.

The key is learning to adapt to natural changes as they happen, rather than fighting them or dreading them. This takes an element of positivity in your outlook, but more than that, it takes faith in yourself and in the people around you that you will all make the changes work and find the good in them. It also takes great faith in God; trusting that there is a plan to bring us to a stronger, happier place.

King Saul is an example of a man fighting changes when he needed to adapt and trust in God. He was a good leader for a long time. He, with the advice of his mentor Samuel, brought freedom and positive changes for his people. However, after many years, he began to ignore the advice of Samuel and the voice of God, in favour of what he wanted. In 1 Samuel 15:2-3 (NLT), Samuel told Saul, *'This is what the LORD of Heaven's Armies has declared: I have decided to settle accounts with the nation of Amalek for opposing Israel when they came from Egypt. ³Now go and completely destroy the entire Amalekite nation— men, women, children, babies, cattle, sheep, goats, camels, and donkeys.'*

Saul took his men and indeed destroyed the Amalekites, but with a few exceptions. He captured their King instead of killing him, and Saul and his men took all the best livestock for themselves. This led God to tell Samuel, *'I am sorry that I ever made Saul king, for he has not been loyal to me and has refused to obey my command.'* 1 Samuel 15:11-12 (NLT).

Saul was again faced with a new challenge in the Philistines and their warrior Goliath. Here, he failed to ask Samuel for his advice, again trusting in his own understanding, rather than seeking the wisdom of others in how to best adapt to the situation. In the end, David rose up, bringing the needed change for the Israelites and becoming their new King. If Saul had stopped to listen to those around him and make the necessary changes, he might have held onto his place of leadership, instead of losing it.

So How do We Come to Terms with Change?

Adapt with the change. We can't always change what goes on in the world, but we can control our reactions.

Stay positive. An important thing to remember in the face of change is that new opportunities will always arise. If you are facing a negative change, know a positive one will come along eventually. And with every change in life, there is some good that can come of it. Remember Romans 8:28 (NIV) *We know that in all things God works for the good of those who love him, who have been called according to his purpose.*

Trust that God has a plan. When I am frightened of the new and grieving the old, I am always comforted by knowledge that I was created with a plan for good in God's mind.

Remember that we can grow from difficulty. No one likes change that brings hardships, but there is no denying that they shape us, and if we use these moments to grow, they can make us into stronger people.

Reflection Questions

- What has been a positive change in my past?
- What has been a negative change? What did I learn from it?
- What gives me peace in the face of unknown challenges?
- What behaviours do I need to cease?
- What can I start doing instead?

Behavioural Expression Five:
Displays Resilience

> **H** Attempts to press through life's hard challenges by adapting new capabilities and capacities.
>
> **M** Demonstrates flexibility but under pressure reverts to old habits and practices.
>
> **L** Falters under life's hard challenges without recourse for developing new capabilities and capacities.

Where Can I Grow my Resilience?

Handling Life's Difficulties

Do we face them head-on, or do we tend to procrastinate or simply ignore them? Do challenges make us feel anxious? Depressed? Exhilarated? Angry?

We handle hardships in different ways. Sometimes, we might leap towards challenges, looking forward to the chance to prove ourselves as strong or capable. Sometimes, we approach more cautiously, looking from every perspective before carefully wading into the situation if need be. And sometimes, we feel so overwhelmed by difficulties that it can be hard to get out of bed, much less face the issue. Some problems will feel more overwhelming than others, and almost all of us have, at some point, felt broken, stuck or hopeless in a difficult situation.

Procrastination only moves the problem to a later date and often compounds it. Perhaps there was a speeding fine that we shelved until the fine doubled or a time where we stayed in a miserable job out of fear of quitting and finding something new. Sometimes, we procrastinate because it feels too hard. Sometimes, we want to give up halfway through. Either way, we are struggling with our resilience and finding innovative ways to handle these challenges.

The Temptation to Return to Old Habits

When Moses led the Israelites out of slavery in Egypt—out of an extremely cruel and difficult life—they came to the very edge of the land that God had called them to. The promised land was before them, yet they were too afraid to enter, too afraid of its inhabitants, the uncertainty and the discomfort. This fear, this lack of trust in God, drove them to want to return to Egypt and their former lives of slavery. Instead, they were made to wander the desert for forty years.

It was the next generation of Israelites, those who grew up in the desert, who finally inherited the promised land. This new generation became resilient and innovative, pressing through life's hard challenges and adapting new capabilities and capacities.

Resilience is built in tough times.

Reflection Questions

- How have I dealt with a difficult time in my past? What did I learn from that?
- Where am I facing hardships right now?
- Where do I have opportunities to build resilience?
- What behaviours do I need to cease?
- What can I start doing instead?

Behavioural Expression Six:
Lives with Purpose

H Unwaveringly pursues commitments, responsibilities and goals with focus and without wavering.

M Pursues commitments, responsibility and goals but is hindered by distractions.

L Feels high dissatisfaction. Tends to wander aimlessly and reactively rather than with a focus on achieving goals.

Keeping Focused on Your Purpose

Distraction of Comparison

Even a strong leader who has learnt to adapt to new situations and has built up a strong resilience, can find themselves distracted from their calling. One of the largest distractions is a comparison to those around us. As we all have been called to different assignments, the journey and result will look different for each person.

As an example, let's look at four men from the New Testament: Stephen, Philip, Paul and James. All four were called to share the Gospel of Christ and became major figures in the early Christian movement, yet all had different assignments.

Stephen, filled with the Holy Spirit and wisdom, was empowered to stand before an angry high council and present an account of God's intervention in Israel's history. He finished with accusations of their involvement in Jesus' crucifixion, and as a result, was stoned. The outcome of his death was the spread of Christianity.

> *A great wave of persecution began that day, sweeping over the church in Jerusalem; and all the believers except the apostles were scattered through the regions of Judea and Samaria.*
> Acts 8:1(NLT)

Philip the Evangelist began his journey after he witnessed his friend Stephen's stoning. He is only mentioned a few times in the New Testament, including in Acts 8, where he met and baptised an Ethiopian eunuch. This was the beginning of the Ethiopian church. Philip may not have been an author or a church-planter, and he never reached the fame of Paul, but his role was no less significant.

Paul's clear assignment was to take the gospel to the Gentiles. He planted many churches, and wrote letters of encouragement and exhortation, many of which are included in the New Testament.

And of course, James, the brother of John, who unwaveringly pursued his commitment to God, even at the price of his own life. James was the first of the twelve to be martyred, killed with the sword by order of

King Herod Agrippa I of Judea, about 44 A.D. His role was cut short, yet he still had a place of significance.

Success Comes From Our Assignment

We shouldn't compare these men with one another: while they all spread the Gospel of Christ, each worked and was successful in his own way. Likewise, we must avoid comparing our own assignment/purpose with those of others.

So, what does success look like in our own lives? Culture would have us see success as things like the amount of money we earn, the car we drive, the house we live in, vacations we take, the qualifications we hold... The truth is that our real success comes from being on the journey to accomplish our individual God assignment.

Reflection Questions

- What do I value? What's important? What's my assignment?
- How can I increase my energy and engagement in this assignment?
- Where do I compare my assignment to that of others?
- What behaviours do I need to cease?
- What can I start doing instead?

COMPETENCY FIVE

Reduced Risk

Assesses physical, emotional and spiritual vulnerabilities to minimise harm and maximise safety.

We live in a world of risk, and the more influence we have in our community, the more responsibility we bear to protect those around us from these risks.

Risks can arise from anyone, any situation—from expanding a church by opening a new location, to hiring staff members, to how we choose to spend our private lives... Do you have the financial resources to open a new location? Does this new hire have a Biblical mindset? Are you taking care of your physical and emotional well-being? We must be aware of risks that arise in order to manage and reduce threats to ourselves and our communities.

These behavioural expressions can help you feel more prepared and in control when risk inevitably comes knocking at your door.

Behavioural Expression One:
Responds to Emergencies with Readiness, Calm and Confident Leadership

H Identifies potential dangers, threats, and risks to oneself and others, sounds the safety alarm and formulates contingency courses of action.

M Takes a casual approach to potential dangers, threats and risks, being motivated by fear, passivity or indifference.

L Responds blindly to potential dangers, threats and risks, leading to the failure of prevention or formulating contingency courses of action.

Staying Calm Amongst the Risks

Keeping Calm to Reduce Risks

When we were building our current house, we wanted to be onsite as much as possible, to be part of the process of construction. The builder was a friend of ours and told me that we could come if we got 'the white card.' This is a certificate that identifies a person onsite to be highly visible to others, and therefore, less likely to be injured. It's a way to be extra aware to protect the business, employees and clients.

Identifying Potential Crises

In my experience, this is something that pastors and leaders should pay attention to as well. We need to be able to evaluate our circumstances and assess risk in order to reduce threats. While the threats are often different from those in construction work—less risk of physical injury, for instance—we still need to be aware of the mental and emotional needs of our staff. Often, we prepare ourselves and our teams for the wrong potential crises.

Recognising the Signs of Burnout

When I became a pastor, I thought the biggest dangers were things like being caught up in pride or love of money or immoral relationships, so I did what I could to reduce risks of these dangers. However, I did not consider burnout, and I did not see it coming. Burnout is actually far more common for most professions than any of the dangers I was concerned about.

How to Avoid Burnout?

How can we avoid the unpredictable and the unseen dangers?

Look and plan ahead.

Speak to others more experienced in our field and to well-being mentors/supervisors.

Document areas of risk and warning signs, and build clear procedures to communicate danger and make safe. Warning signs include fatigue, low role clarity, bullying, harassment, even violence or aggression. If there are even subtle hints of these behaviours or miscommunications, they will almost always grow and become more threatening. Think of cars with noises and lights that alert us to all sorts of dangers: unfastened seat belts, unclosed doors, our vehicle getting too close to an object... These are all signs that we need to take action to prevent an accident from happening.

Addressing these potential risks with the person who is giving warning signs can allow the leadership and the individual to be more aware of their motivations and feelings. It is important during these conversations to come from a place of concern and grace, rather than anger or judgement. Otherwise, confronting the problem may lead to a larger one. When a risk does arise (and this can still happen despite healthy work environments) a good leader will approach with calm and confident leadership.

Reflection Questions

- Where are the danger zones in my world?
- How can I prepare or prevent these dangers?
- What is my typical response to dangers? How could I improve?
- What behaviours should I cease? What can I start doing instead?

Behavioural Expression Two:
Implements a Plan for Well-Being

> **H** Practises a strategy that enables work-life and home-life to flourish.
>
> **M** Yearns for work-life and home-life to flourish but fails to implement a strategy for flourishing.
>
> **L** Practises no strategy that enables work-life and home-life to flourish.

Planning for Being Well, Requires a Plan for Well-Being

Myth: If they are doing God's will, the staff won't get physically or emotionally sick.

Myth: We don't need to look after them, that's God's job.

Debunked: Paul the apostle stated that his ministry to the Galatian church commenced when he was sick, and he was looked after by them.

> *Surely you remember that I was sick when I first brought you the Good News. But even though my condition tempted you to reject me, you did not despise me or turn me away. You took me in and cared for me as though I were an angel from God or even Christ Jesus himself.*
> Galatians 4:13, 14 (NLT)

We need to allocate enough resources to ensure well-being. Yes, both time and money.

$30 Expense or $2000 Bill Your Choice

Often the perception is that we don't have the resources to properly take care of ourselves and those around us. This is both naïve and irresponsible. If you don't work on ensuring well-being, you will pay a bigger cost later. It's like servicing a car: you can get away without doing maintenance for a while, but you will eventually pay a bigger price. I have a ride-on lawnmower that I purchased second-hand. It went well, and not understanding that I needed to look after the oil level and oblivious to the motor's health, I kept on mowing until there was a loud bang and the motor stopped. The motor had to be replaced. A little time checking and adding 5 litres of oil for $30 would have saved me $2000 for a new motor. This was an expensive lesson.

I met with two pastors who were chatting about the huge amount of time they had invested in a church and its leadership to help it through a crisis after the pastor had fallen morally. They were called in along with others to assist and help the church recover. Crisis care like this is costly in time, money and energy, not only for the new pastors, but also for the entire church team.

It's a true statement that the health of the leader impacts the health of an organisation. When a leader becomes burnt out, the whole enterprise suffers. This usually shows in the bottom line—money decreases (some cases by over 50%) and key people leave. Could your organisation afford to have over 50% decrease in income?

Coming Home From Work Healthy and Safe

What is your board's/employer's plan for your well-being? Is it clear and functional? If you are a sole operator/director, what is your well-being plan? What are you doing to ensure that your employee's well-being is looked after?

This means that as an employer, you must pay attention to risks both physical and emotional, and address these concerns well before they become an emergency. For example, are you providing enough time off and encouraging employees to set healthy work-life boundaries before burnout occurs. A good employer takes preventative steps to avoid even early stages of declining health.

It is wonderful to see a growing focus on developing a workplace mental health strategy. Does your board have a strategy for the well-being of its employees? Under Australian Work Health and Safety (WHS) legislation, employers must take steps to protect workers against risks to their physical and mental health.

New Zealand also has legislation in place for the psychological well-being of employees. Worksafe's article on health is very clear that the focus is not just physical. Furthermore, the Persons Conducting a Business or Undertaking have a primary duty to care for their workers. I love the NZ Worksafe vision that by 2026 'Everyone who goes to work comes home healthy and safe.'

Where Are You Most at Risk?

Board directors and decision-makers have an obligation to ensure the health and safety of workers engaged in the business. Safe Work Australia says, 'This includes taking reasonable steps to gain an understanding of the psychosocial hazards and risks associated with the operations of the business or undertaking, and to ensure the business or undertaking has and uses appropriate resources and processes to eliminate or minimise risks to psychological health.'

It is advised that boards prepare and implement a strategy for the well-being of their key employees. What is the first concern on the list of causes of psychological injury for Christian leaders? Psychological damage. A study from the *Research Insights from the Flourishing in Ministry Project* has found that 40% of pastors report stress due to significant workloads. In the same article, The United Methodist Church worked with Dr Deshon, a leading expert on job analysis, to understand why so many members of their clergy experience high stress. Dr Deshon determined that to perform all their tasks effectively would require 64 different personal competencies. He concluded that 'it is almost inconceivable to imagine that a single person could be uniformly high on the sixty-four distinct knowledge, skills, abilities, and personal characteristics.' For more information on stresses in ministry, you can read the entire article at https://workwellresearch.com/media/images/FIM%20Report%20Workload.pdf

People in ministry need more support and more protection than they are receiving.

What Are Your Jurisdiction's Responsibilities?

Surely, for those of us who are Christ-followers, there is a greater reason and responsibility to prevent harm, intervene early and support recovery. As Paul says in Galatians 6:10 (NLT) *Therefore, whenever we have the opportunity, we should do good to everyone—especially to those in the family of faith.*

Reflection Questions

- What are my workplace responsibilities for well-being?
- Where are the hazards to be aware of in my life?
- What behaviours do I need to cease?
- What can I start doing instead?

Behavioural Expression Three:
Engages in Accountable Relationships

H Actively utilises 360-degree feedback to gain self-insight. Welcomes a mentor's discernment, feedback and coaching.

M Discloses selectively and cautiously. May battle with rejection and trust.

L Avoids consultation and disclosure with professionals, medical doctors and peers.

360-Degree Care

We recognize the need for medical doctors to tell us what is wrong because we simply can't always know what is going on inside of us. We have regular checkups, take medication if we need to, and follow the advice of health-care professionals.

For some reason, we treat our mental and emotional health very differently from our physical health. When we are experiencing these kinds of issues, many of us try to fix them ourselves, or perhaps just shove them down and ignore them. Truthfully, no one can manage all their mental and emotional issues on their own. Many of us seek the help of a therapist, a mentor or a coach in much the same way we consult a medical doctor. Even if we don't see a professional, we rely on the people close to us to discuss and reflect on our mental and emotional health to provide new insight for us and help us work through problems.

360-Degree Approach

I like to take what I call the 360-degree approach to gain insight. I look above, below and alongside—meaning I look to the people with more experience and wisdom than I have (mentors, supervisors), I look to the people with less experience for whom I bear some responsibility (mentees, employees) and I look alongside me at people I consider peers (friends, family). I make sure to position myself to be able to listen to feedback and be able to trust the relationship so that I am not guarded or hostile. This way I can feel certain that I have seen myself from many different perspectives and can then use this information and assistance to create a strategy for my sustainable well-being.

Having these people involved in your world is so important to help see areas of vulnerability and areas of risk where you aren't thriving.

Reflection Questions

- Who can I go to for honest and open feedback?
- Who is helping me care for my soul, mind and heart?
- What behaviours do I need to cease?
- What can I start doing instead?

Behavioural Expression Four:
Creates Margins in Life

- **H** Generates surplus capacity for the unexpected in all areas of life.
- **M** Makes allowances for abnormal circumstances but at times compromises boundaries and depletes personal resources.
- **L** Maintains no latitude for life's difficulties. Often finds it difficult to say 'no'.

No one likes to think about the worst-case scenarios in our lives, and even less, do we like to plan for them. It can feel negative, faithless, overly cautious and unnecessary. But it is necessary. We don't need to live in fear, but adding some margin for catastrophe in our lives can help us to feel safe and in control of our own futures.

Look at your life. Do you have the capacity to weather a storm? Are you planning for the unexpected?

Differentiating the Margins of Life

We need margins in many areas: physical, financial, and emotional.

Physically, we need to give our bodies a margin; are we doing well in caring for our bodies so they can withstand sickness? A night of poor sleep? A morning of intense exercise? What happens when your body goes through something serious? Are you able to take the time needed to rest and replenish?

Financially, do you have enough saved for car troubles? Health scares? What if you lose your job? What is your safety net?

And finally, there are the often-neglected, emotional margins. Are you giving yourself the outlets you need? Can you process feelings as they happen instead of letting them build? Are you making sure you give yourself time for fun, relaxation and relationships? Do you have enough in your tank to handle an emotionally stressful situation?

We need these margins not only for ourselves, but also to be able to help the people around us. We want to be able to intervene or be of assistance when there is an opportunity. This is only possible if we are taking care of ourselves and building up healthy margins that allow us space, time and resources to then help others.

Reflection Questions

- What can I do to increase margins?
- How do I successfully prepare for the unexpected?
- Do I have enough buoyancy to survive the unexpected?
- What behaviours do I need to cease?
- What can I start doing instead?

Conclusion

What happens now? You have come this far; you have explored each competency of a healthy Christian leader and you have reflected on their behavioural expressions. Hopefully you have been sharing your reflections with a mentor and gaining new insights from their perspective while also asking the Lord for transformation as you read and reflect.

What have you learnt during this journey? What have you uncovered about yourself, your relationships, your goals and your motivations? Take a few minutes to look back on each of the five core competencies and recall the feelings and revelation that arose as you learnt about each of them.

Vital Spirituality Has an intimate relationship with God that is life changing and life giving.

Thriving Relationships Demonstrates an understanding of others and intentionally develops and maintains close connections.

Emotional Intelligence Uses empathy and wisdom while navigating relationships and difficult situations.

Sustainable Life Takes actions and forms behaviours that enhance long-term viability and overall health.

Reduced Risk Assesses physical, emotional and spiritual vulnerabilities to minimise harm and maximise safety for themselves and those around them.

Which competency was the most difficult for you? Which felt natural and easy to consider? Which competency needs more development?

If you are still struggling to answer these questions, this is a great opportunity to turn to your mentor or find a mentor if you don't have one. We have found that engaging a mentor helps to add accountability and can help you to understand what is happening in you. You go to a doctor because you want to live a physically well life, not just because you need to recover. A mentor can help you avoid or handle burnout and trauma. They can help you live a fulfilled and resilient life, not being impaired by a poor vision for health.

God didn't mean for us to walk this world alone, nor are we meant to understand who we are and our purpose without the help of others.

Final Reflection

- Where have I grown?
- What will help me maintain this health?
- During my reading of this book, what changes have I noticed in my life?
- What do I want to change, where do I want to increase health?
- Who's going to help me achieve this change?

APPENDIX

Health of a Christian Leader Assessment

Competency One: Vital Spirituality

Behavioural Expression 1:
Aligns identity in Christ with scripture.

H Shares energetically with others what God is saying and routinely implements his precepts from scriptures into one's personal identity and actions.

M Senses God's voice occasionally when reading scriptures, which results in modest impact on one's personal identity and actions.

L Practises religious rituals and reads scripture as duty, but finds it dull, with no sense of God's precepts from scriptures impacting one's personal identity and actions.

Behavioural Expression 2:
Engages in a rich prayer life.

H Talks with God unceasingly regardless of life circumstances and looks for opportunities to similarly pray with others.

M Talks with God regularly and occasionally prays with others.

L Prays infrequently.

Behavioural Expression 3:
Experiences God's involvement in all areas of life.

H Confidently shares past and present experiences of God's involvement in one's thoughts, conversations, and events.

M Identifies personal encounters and experiences of God but struggles to recognise God's present involvement in one's thoughts, conversations, and events.

L Has limited or no sense of God's involvement in one's personal life.

Behavioural Expression 4:
Exhibits a transformative connection with God.

H Maintains an intimate relationship with God, resulting in continual spiritual and personal growth.

M Knows God personally but without close intimacy, resulting in stagnation of spiritual and personal growth.

L Stays feeling disconnected from God. May be failing to resist personal temptations.

Competency Two: Thriving Relationships

Behavioural Expression 1:
Builds secure attachments.

- **H** Promotes a deep sense of contentment and belonging in relationships.
- **M** Connects well, but may allow insecurities to cause either some detachment or controlling of relationships.
- **L** Perpetuates either high detachment or toxic dependence in relationships.

Behavioural Expression 2:
Adapts to improve meaningful connection with others.

- **H** Exhibits flexibility, while affirming deep, accountable connections, during changing circumstances.
- **M** Endeavours to live in harmony with others, but too easily avoids efforts to resolve difficult problems with interpersonal relationships.
- **L** Exacerbates interpersonal problems with people through personal rigidity or provocation.

Behavioural Expression 3:
Communicates transparently, effectively, and wisely.

- **H** Builds trust through active and compassionate listening, articulating clearly, and showing vulnerability.

- **M** Facilitates free-flowing communication, but allows fear of rejection to cause limited transparency.

- **L** Focuses and redirects conversations constantly on oneself or resorts to silence when one's voice needs to be heard.

Behavioural Expression 4:
Manages conflict well.

- **H** Seeks understanding of critical issues without attacking persons and assertively seeks resolution without aggression.

- **M** Shows courage to resolve misunderstandings but tends to personalise rather then objectify critical issues. Does not usually express one's own needs or feelings.

- **L** Avoids conflict whenever possible and capitulates to its consequences. May become emotionally volatile when confronted about critical issues.

Behavioural Expression 5:
Demonstrates Forgiveness.

- **H** Releases others graciously from their wrongdoings.
- **M** Maintains some grudges when feeling justified.
- **L** Recounts others' wrongs readily, and cuts offenders from key relationships.

Competency Three: Emotional Intelligence

Behavioural Expression 1:
Grows in self-awareness.

- **H** Continually evaluates oneself honestly, despite seeing undesirable aspects of the self-picture.
- **M** Reacts to, rather than endeavours to understand, emotional and physical distress.
- **L** Fails to recognise or give space to emotions and related physical reactions.

Behavioural Expression 2:
Practises self-reflection.

- **H** Sets aside regular time for self-reflection and acts on constructive insights gained.
- **M** Increases in understanding of emotional blind spots and their physical effect but without acting accordingly.
- **L** Gives little to no time to the habit of self-reflection.

Behavioural Expression 3:
Maintains emotional well-being.

- **H** Displays energy for life, love and work, and assists others in making changes in their lives.
- **M** Stays afloat during the normal challenges of life but falters in a crisis.
- **L** Stays in a state of emotional emptiness. May be accompanied by fatigue, numbness, and ineffective decision-making.

Behavioural Expression 4:
Cultivates a Biblical mindset.

H Filters attitudes and perspectives through scriptural principles rather than humanistic attitudes and perspectives.

M Endeavours to filter attitudes and perspectives through scriptural principles, but allows negativity to cause self-doubt and indecision.

L Anticipates and finds negativity constantly without filtering attitudes and perspectives through Godly principles.

Behavioural Expression 5:
Self-regulates emotions.

H Behaves responsibly toward oneself and others regardless of one's momentary feelings.

M Forgoes restraint when feeling uncertain or threatened.

L Reacts without restraint and regard to the impact of one's reaction on self and others.

Behavioural Expression 6:
Displays humility.

- **H** Demonstrates a modest view of oneself as evidenced through altruism, empathy and curiosity to learn.
- **M** Displays appreciation of others' strengths and contributions but under pressure becomes closed-minded and thinks one knows best.
- **L** Tends to find solutions alone, perceives that one's own ability is superior, and resists constructive feedback.

Competency Four: Sustainable Life

Behavioural Expression 1:
Maintains self-control.

- **H** Makes responsible choices based on sound judgement while keeping one's impulses under control.
- **M** Relinquishes sound judgement under pain or pressure, resulting in diminished disciplines.
- **L** Displays unsound judgement routinely through compulsive actions or impulsive choices.

Behavioural Expression 2:
Manages stress.

H Develops awareness of stress and is proactive in mitigating its effects.

M Shows an inability sometimes to set boundaries and allows unnecessary stress to accumulate.

L Disregards stress level and over-exerts to the point of experiencing physical symptoms.

Behavioural Expression 3:
Demonstrates personal responsibility.

H Takes ownership for the consequences of one's actions rather than blaming other people or circumstances.

M Tends to self-isolate and problem solve alone when consultation with and support from others is warranted.

L Takes no ownership for the consequences of one's actions and blames other people or circumstances.

Behavioural Expression 4:
Embraces necessary change.

H Finds innovative solutions and makes changes when needed, even when changing is difficult.

M Makes some constructive changes but often reactively rather than proactively.

L Stays stuck in unproductive patterns, habits, and commitments.

Behavioural Expression 5:
Displays resilience.

- **H** Attempts to press through life's hard challenges by adapting new capabilities and capacities.
- **M** Demonstrates flexibility but under pressure reverts to old habits and practices.
- **L** Falters under life's hard challenges without recourse for developing new capabilities and capacities.

Behavioural Expression 6:
Lives with purpose.

- **H** Unwaveringly pursues commitments, responsibilities and goals with focus and without wavering.
- **M** Pursues commitments, responsibilities, and goals but gets hindered by distractions.
- **L** Feels high dissatisfaction. Tends to wander aimlessly and reactively rather than with a focus on achieving goals.

Competency Five: Reduced Risk

Behavioural Expression 1:
Responds to emergencies with readiness, calm and confident leadership.

- **H** Identifies potential dangers, threats, and risks to oneself and others, sounds the safety alarm and formulates contingency courses of action.

- **M** Takes a casual approach to potential dangers, threats, and risks being motivated by fear, passivity, or indifference.

- **L** Responds blindly to potential dangers, threats, and risks, leading to the failure at prevention or formulating contingency courses of action.

Behavioural Expression 2:
Implements a plan for well-being.

- **H** Practises a strategy that enables work-life and home-life to flourish.

- **M** Yearns for work-life and home-life to flourish but fails to implement a strategy for flourishing.

- **L** Practises no strategy that enables work-life and home-life to flourish.

Behavioural Expression 3:
Engages in accountable relationships.

- **H** Actively utilises 360-degree feedback to gain self-insight. Welcomes a mentor's discernment, feedback and coaching.
- **M** Discloses selectively and cautiously. May battle with rejection and trust.
- **L** Avoids consultation and disclosure with professionals, medical doctors and peers.

Behavioural Expression 4:
Creates margins in life.

- **H** Generates surplus capacity for the unexpected in all areas of life.
- **M** Makes allowances for abnormal circumstances but at times compromises boundaries and depletes personal resources.
- **L** Maintains no latitude for life's difficulties. Often finds it difficult to say 'no'.

Author Bio

Dr Don Easton's passion is to lift the buoyancy and resilience of Christian leaders to enhance the well-being, sustainability, and safety of communities.

After journeying through severe burnout in 2014, he has conducted qualitative research to quantify ideal Christian leader health and develop pathways to well-being. This outfits him to build resilience and aid revitalisation.

Don founded Verve Lead to develop and multiply quality well-being mentors.

The Verve Lead team consults with movements, develops mentors and provides mentoring and professional supervision to executive, global and local Christian leaders.

Don's forty-seven years of ministry experience includes church planting and ordained ministry in traditional and Pentecostal churches. His roles as Senior Minister for thirty-one years and on a national executive for ten years position him to understand the complexities and pressures of ministry.

His life experience and formal education have equipped him as a Well-being Mentor, Professional Supervisor and Consultant.

Also by Dr Don Easton

BURNOUT & BEYOND

The Dangers of Depletion and the Path to Health

Praise for Burnout and Beyond

"Don has done the difficult, personal work of recovery and has created a sustainable rhythm to avoid repeating burnout in his own life. He has also done the hard work of research and professional growth to become a leading voice in his culture and times. Don has years of rich experience in leading other clergy into healthier, sustainable rhythms. Like all great pastors, Don has synthesised complex scholarship, life and ministry leadership experience, and Biblical and theological principles to create a contextualised, practical resource accessible to all. This resource is especially timely given the impact of ministry stress during the global pandemic and whatever the new normal looks like for clergy. Don artfully dispels some of the common myths of ministry burnout and provides invaluable insights and practical advice that can keep pastors from being blindsided and impaired. May our Lord Jesus Christ restore the joy of your salvation and the joy of ministry as you implement the recommended practices in the pages that follow."

Rev. Christopher J. Adams, PhD.

"Don has written with honesty, courage and humility, addressing the issue of emotional depletion and burnout at a time when pastors are being affected in unprecedented numbers.

It has been a privilege to support Don as a mentor for about 8 years, and to rejoice at his recaptured health, vitality and passion to help other pastors.

The gauges he presents are particularly helpful for anyone seeking to recover from emotional depletion.

I highly recommend this excellent book."

Dr. Keith Farmer

Mentor, Principal Emeritus, Australian College of Ministries. Doctor of Ministry, Fuller Theological Seminary.

"My friend Don has faithfully served as senior minister with C3 Global for over 30 years and sharing from his own journey brings a book that will help so many. Burnout is a significant problem today. Don's book helps us understand the problem and gives pathways to recover and thrive again. He gives us good news that we can get through whatever we face."

Ps Dr Phil Pringle AOM

Global President C3 Church

"Burnout and meltdowns seem to be the lot of producers; they simply don't know when or even how to stop, much less listen. I'm not sure Don's sage advice (and it is certainly worth listening to) will stop the process, but what he has written will definitely help you navigate your way out, and, in his parlance, find a richer and more enduring future – something he is now enjoying.

Don has disarmingly invited us to the inner workings and processing of a very painful time in his life. His honesty is the first step to healing, his willingness to listen the second, and his self-awareness the key to maintaining a healthy, less driven, and fulfilling lifestyle. He shows that there is light on the other side of darkness.

The text is full of wise advice, helpful steps, and excellent resources. Don writes to all situations, having read and studied widely, and not that of his profession only. As you read, I'm sure you'll be confronted, challenged and thereby changed – hopefully.

I unreservedly recommend Dr Don Easton's story to you."

Simon McIntyre
C3 Church Global Team; Americas

"The pressures and challenges of leadership contribute directly to the increasing stories of adrenaline exhaustion and burnout. In this excellent book, Don shares his own story with great courage and vulnerability, offering us much needed wisdom and many practical insights for staying healthy over the long haul. Highly recommended."

Dr Mark Conner

Speaker, Author, Trainer, Coach

"It has been a pleasure working with Don over the past few years. Following his studies at Fuller, he brought back considerable expertise in mentoring people to avoid burnout and stay true to mission. We have been so impressed by his expertise that a wide selection of our senior staff consult regularly with him as part of keeping their professional, spiritual and family life on track. This has now continued for a number of years and is a testimony to his theoretical knowledge, practical knowledge and expertise. All professionals in the ministry will benefit from engaging with Don and his work."

Rees Davis

Executive Principal, King's Christian College

"When you are going through any kind of crisis the best person to look to is one who has been there, done that and survived! Don Easton's book Burnout and Beyond draws from the wellspring of his own personal journey through burnout to recovery. Don humbly describes the subtle and gradual nature of his decline into the valley, the challenges and struggles back to a place of healing and restoration, and the deep lessons learned along the way.

This book outlines clearly the deep causes of burnout and its symptoms. It also gives real tools for evaluating your emotional health and wellbeing and outlines some very sound and practical steps for a holistic approach to recovery. Best of all it gives hope that burnout is not "the end destination but can be a path to a better, stronger you." If you have experienced the pain of burnout, feel like you are heading towards it, or simply want to avoid it altogether, Don's book will prove invaluable."

Ps Wayne Peat
Coordinator C3 Pacific Pastor's Support

"In all my years of ministry I'm not sure I can recall a time when I sensed that so many leaders/ministers were feeling weary, under pressure and certainly a lot less motivated than they would hope to be. So, to say that Don's book is timely is an understatement.

When I reconnected with Don a few years ago I was struck by the deep peace, humility and calmness in his life. Yes, he's walked the path of burnout, but he has also slowly and intentionally walked the path of healing too.

I encourage leaders to read this book and grasp the invaluable wisdom and practical insight–but most importantly–I encourage leaders to read this inspirational story of truth, hope, recovery–and above all the grace of our wonderful God."

Rev Dr Graham Humphris
Chairperson Generate Presbytery UCASA

"In Burnout & Beyond Don Easton shares vulnerably about his personal journey of burnout and recovery. This book is filled with practical, research-based solutions to help guide you to a place of better health. It is a must-read for anyone living with high demands."

John Finkelde

Founder, Grow a Healthy Church

"In his book Burnout and Beyond, Don Easton provides us with an insightful and practical guide for identifying, dealing with and discovering wholeness in his journey with burnout. He combines this with some very helpful professional guidelines as well."

I highly recommend this book to anyone experiencing burnout and also to leaders, family, professionals and associates in order to gain a greater understanding of burnout and the way forward to healing and wholeness."

REFERENCES

Adams, C., Bloom, M. (2017) Flourishing in Ministry: Wellbeing at Work in Helping Professions. *Journal of Psychology and Christianity*, vol. 36. 254–258, https://doi.org/https://www.crcna.org/sites/default/files/adams_bloom_jpc_fall_2017_article.pdf.

Bloom, M. (2017) *A Burden Too Heavy? Research Insights from the Flourishing in Ministry Project*. University of Notre Dame.

Bradberry, T., Greaves, J. (2009) *Emotional Intelligence 2.0*. TalentSmart.

Community Driver Reviver. *NSW*, (2021.11.12) http://roadsafety.transport.nsw.gov.au/stayingsafe/fatigue/driverreviver/index.html.

Covey, Stephen R. (2012) *Wisdom and Teachings of Stephen R. Covey*. Simon & Schuster Ltd.

Encyclopedia Britannica, (1998.07.20) Protestant Ethic https://www.britannica.com/topic/Protestant-ethic.

George, Carl F. (2017) *How to Break Growth Barriers: Revise Your Role, Release Your People, and Capture Overlooked Opportunities for Your Church*. Baker Book House.

Hart, A.D. (1995) *The Hidden Link between Adrenalin & Stress: The Exciting New Breakthrough That Helps You Overcome Stress Damage*. Kindle Edition ed., Thomas Nelson.

Hart, A.D., and May, S. (2003) *Safe Haven Marriage: A Marriage You Can Come Home To*. Thomas Nelson.

Hybels, B. (2012) *Courageous Leadership*. Zondervan.

Lencioni, P. M. (2007) *The Five Dysfunctions of a Team: A Leadership Fable*. Enhanced Edition ed., John Wiley & Sons.

Lewis, R. (2009) *Mentoring Matters*, Monarch Books, Grand Rapids, MI. 183

List of Fatal Snake Bites in Australia (2021.10.09) In *Wikipedia*, https://en.wikipedia.org/wiki/List_of_fatal_snake_bites_in_Australia.

Moore, G. (2015) *Going to the Next Level*. Ark House Press.

Pape, S. (2022) *The Barefoot Investor: The Only Money Guide You'll Ever Need*. Wiley. Kindle Edition.

Proeschold-Bell, R. J. (2012.07) An Overview of the History and Current Status of Clergy Health, Duke Global Health Institute. https://www.researchgate.net/publication/225305911_An_Overview_of_the_History_and_Current_Status_of_Clergy_Health

Proeschold-Bell, R.J., et al. (2013.08.22) Using Effort-Reward Imbalance Theory to Understand High Rates of Depression and Anxiety among Clergy. https://divinity.duke.edu/sites/divinity.duke.edu/files/documents/chi/Clergy%20Depression%20%26%20Anxiety%20Effort-Reward%20Imbalance_formatted%20for%20web.pdf

Proeschold-Bell, R., et al. "The Glory of God Is a Human Being Fully Alive: Predictors of Positive versus Negative Mental Health among Clergy." *Journal for the Scientific Study of Religion*, vol. 54, no. 4, 2015, 702–721. https://doi.org/10.1111/jssr.12234.

Safework Australia. (2019.01.01) Related Psychological Health and Safety: A Systematic Approach to Meeting Your Duties. *safeworkaustralia.gov.au/Topic/Mental-Health* https://www.safeworkaustralia.gov.au/doc/work-related-psychological-health-and-safety-systematic-approach-meeting-your-duties.

Riley,P., and Sioau-Mai, S. (2020.02) The Australian Principal, Occupational Health, Safety and Wellbeing Survey. *Health and Wellbeing.org*, Institute for Positive Psychology and Education Australian Catholic University. https://www.healthandwellbeing.org/reports/AU/2019%20ACU%20Australian%20Principals%20Report.pdf.

The Rolling Stones (1965) (I Can't Get No) Satisfaction. *On Air*.

Tony Cooke Ministries (2020.12.08) Job Description for Church Staff http://www.tonycooke.org/stories-and-illustrations/job_description/.

Seppälä, E., Moeller, J. 1 (2018.05.16) 1 in 5 Employees Is Highly Engaged and at Risk of Burnout. *Harvard Business Review*. https://hbr.org/2018/02/1-in-5-highly-engaged-employees-is-at-risk-of-burnout.

Siegel, D. (2021.04.18) The Developing Mind: How Relationships and the Brain Interact to Shape Who We Are. Second Edition. https://drdansiegel.com/.

Valcour, M. (2021.08.27) 4 Steps to Beating Burnout. *Harvard Business Review*. https://hbr.org/2016/11/beating-burnout.

Vasagar, J. (2013.08.30) Out of Hours Working Banned by German Labour Ministry. *The Telegraph*, Telegraph Media Group. http://www.telegraph.co.uk/news/worldnews/europe/germany/10276815/Out-of-hours-working-banned-by-German-labour-ministry

World Health Organization (2019.05.28) Burn-out: an Occupational Phenomenon: International Classification of Diseases. https://www.who.int/news/item/28-05-2019-burn-out-an-occupational-phenomenon-international-classification-of-diseases.

www.ingramcontent.com/pod-product-compliance
Lightning Source LLC
Chambersburg PA
CBHW071710020426
42333CB00017B/2213